"History is not just stone, notable people, and bricks.
It includes the reaction of those who were there and
the community's ongoing response."
—Jim Boles

Vanishing Past Series

This book is #4 of the Vanishing Past Series published
by Vanishing Past Press LLC. Vanishing Past Press
is dedicated to the documentation, preservation,
and distribution of works of scholarship and cultural
importance with emphasis on under-examined or
unexplored topics.

This book is part of that effort.

They Did No Harm

Alternative Medicine in Niagara Falls, NY

1830–1930

James M. Boles, Ed.D.

Editor's Note: The exact language of this time has been retained for historical accuracy. No offense is intended toward any individual or group.

Design by: Rachel Bridges Design
Technical Advisor: Carolyn Ryder

ISBN: 978-1-949860-03-0

978-1-949860-03-0

Cover image: Monteagle Hotel, from the Illustrated London News, Vol. 43, no. 1218, p. 193, August 22, 1863

ALWAYS REMEMBER:

"The past is a foreign country: they do things differently there" -L.P. Hartley

Table of Contents

Introduction

While researching early human service agencies in Niagara County New York, I came across a number of healing facilities that did not fit the material that was eventually published in the book, *When There Were Poor Houses*. These commercial ventures were often based upon an alternative view of health care that differed from the traditional care that was available during 1830–1930. In the same period, health products ranging from medicinal mineral waters, patent medicines, food products, and devices were developing in Niagara Falls and many were sold all over the world.

This was in contrast to the medicine practiced at the time, which was largely guesswork and often employed dangerous procedures and risky surgery. In the 1800s and into the early 1900s, medicine was primitive. Physicians often were untrained, and licensing was not yet organized. Bleeding, mercury, and surgeries were the primary methods of treatment. Many died because of this care, and people had little confidence in doctors. Established treatments for people with disabilities were crude and seldom effective, so the sanitariums and alternative methods and products were also used to treat diseases of the nervous system and physical and mental disabilities.

With good marketing and common wisdom, these enterprises used a variety of colorful remedies, often harmless, to help their customers. Mainstream medicine at the time was far more dangerous.

CHAPTER 1

The Medicinal Mineral
Water Hotels

R esearch and reading about mineral springs in the eastern United States shows a pattern of discovery by early travelers and settlers, and their reports often mention the local Native Americans using the springs for medicinal purposes. Springs were clear water or mineral springs. The mineral spring generally had a smell and taste that was different from clear water, and this was an early indication that the spring was a mineral spring. Once the spring was known as a mineral spring, local residents would use the waters to cure their medical problems because medicine of the times had little to offer. Soon businessmen would have the spring analyzed and would commercialize the spring and begin bottling and selling the water and/or building a sanitarium. The facility would then attract tourists and soon after the very ill and invalids, all searching for a cure from this new mineral spring with its claims for healing. When a new spring was discovered and the results of an analysis publicized, the reaction was very similar to the announcement of a new cure or wonder drug for an illness in today's medical world.

The Bellevue/Suspension Bridge section of what is now Niagara Falls contained many springs, both clear and mineral. A short time after the arrival of early white settlers the springs were commercialized utilizing the water to bottle and establish mineral baths and mineral spring hotels.

This group of Niagara Falls health-care facilities, the Medicinal Mineral Water Hotels, used mineral water that was analyzed and specifically used to cure their clients' problems. The hotel names were often confusing. Many were nothing more than hotels with add-ons such as diet, fresh air, and special water baths. They were often focused upon a specific disease or disability, utilizing mineral waters, patent medicines, health foods, and devices available at the time.

The Springs of Suspension Bridge, NY

The springs that were found around the Suspension Bridge area of Niagara Falls appeared to be surfacing in or above the Lockport Dolomite. Ground water is able to flow through this layer and the above layer of sediments but unable to travel through the underlying shale layer (due to physical properties of the lower lying shale). As the water is in the rock layer it dissolves minerals in the rock, giving the water its mineral content.

The nature of ground water is that it flows from areas of high to low pressure and where pressure is not a large factor it flows to the areas of lowest elevation. These features were found in the Monteagle Ridge area of the gorge and at several other areas in the Gorge. As a result, we see the presence of the springs.

The Bellevue Mineral Springs and Bath House at Belle Vue de la Cataracte

This area of today's Niagara Falls was originally known as the Village of Bellevue. The land was along the Niagara River giving a beautiful view of the Cataracts at Niagara Falls. The name was derived from the Bellevue Land Company, the former owners of the property. Before merging with Niagara Falls in 1892, the area was also known as Suspension Bridge.

There were many springs in the village of Bellevue, and there is evidence of use by Native Americans. Bellevue Avenue in the City of Niagara Falls is a historical reminder of the

> The mineral spring at Niagara Falls bids fair to become a place of much resort by the fashionables and invalids. It commands a fine view of the cataract, and its waters prove an efficacious remedy in some disease.

Geneva Gazette, Wednesday, June 15, 1827.

Here is the celebrated

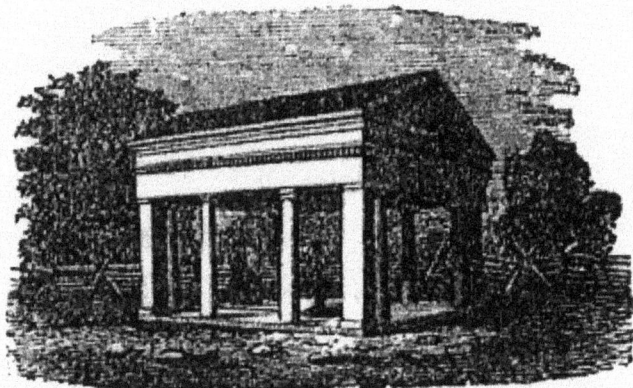

MINERAL SPRING,

"Near the Suspension Bridge is the 'Mineral Spring', welling up among the rocks, into a stone basin. The water is strongly impregnated with sulphur, and contains also lime and magnesia. A chaste little temple covers this famous Spring."

Burke's descriptive guide, 1850.

old name for the area, and Bath and Spring streets refer to the Mineral Springs that were once commercialized by local businessmen.

Early accounts of an undeveloped spring appear on maps of the area on the property of Orson Childs.

The property was improved by Benjamin Rathbun who built the temple over the spring. Further development included a hotel and bath house; the Bellevue Bath house was the first commercial use of the Sulphur Spring.

The medicinal qualities of the water of the Belle Vue Spring are sulphurous; and several well authenticated cures have been effected in the following named diseases: ERYSIPELAS, PILES, RHEUMATISM, ULCEROUS SORES, Decline and general prostration of health, Cutaneous affections, and as a cosmetic it stands very high.

The water is of the description of the Harrowgate, of England, and the White Sulphur, of Virginia. Gentlemen of the medical faculty give it a high recommendation; and for the simple purposes of the bath, both for the sick and well, it is much superior to common water. A commodious Bathing House is established at the Spring which is much resorted to by travelers and by the people of the surrounding country.

Traveler's Guide, 1844

An early traveler's account of the Bellevue Mineral Springs and health benefits.

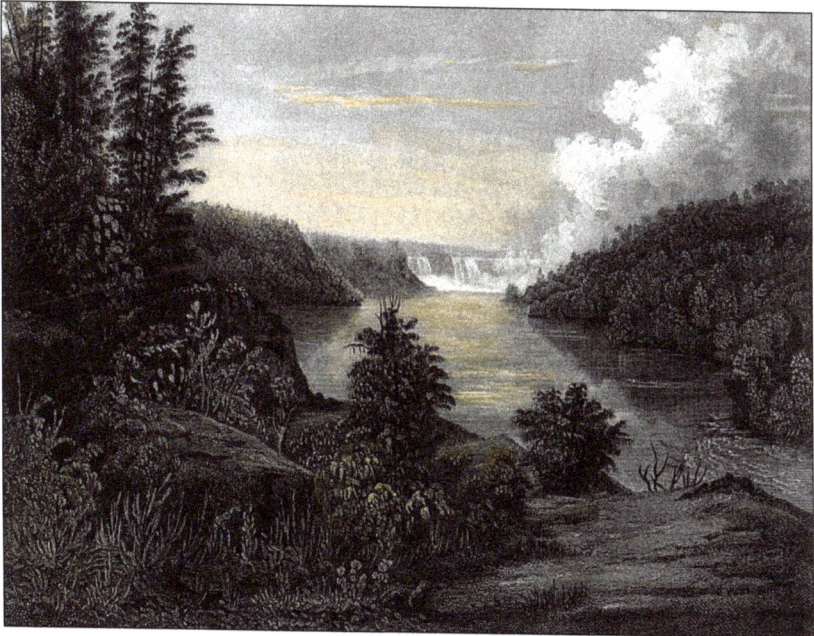

Bellevue Spring Landing on the Niagara River Gorge showing a view of Niagara Falls. From *Ladies' Repository*, Cincinnati and New York, 1848.

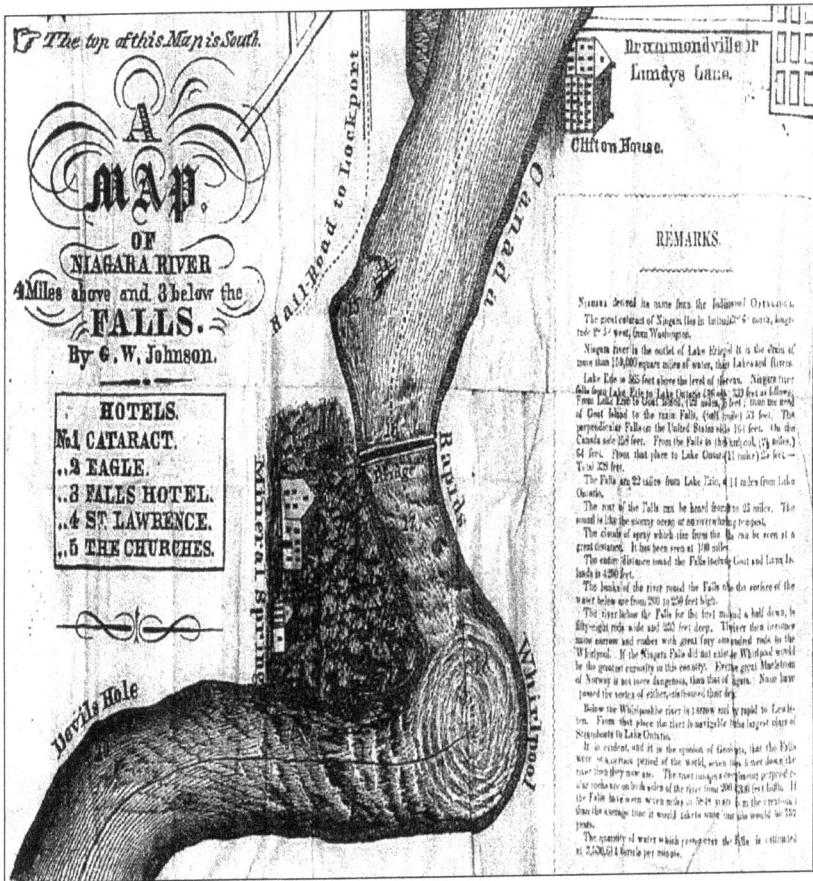

An 1849 map of Niagara Falls, NY, showing the location of the Bellevue Mineral Spring.

The Bellevue Mineral Spring was one of the springs used to supply the nearby Monteagle House with mineral water. This area was near the Old Suspension Bridge with the Spirella Company and the existing United States Customs building close by.

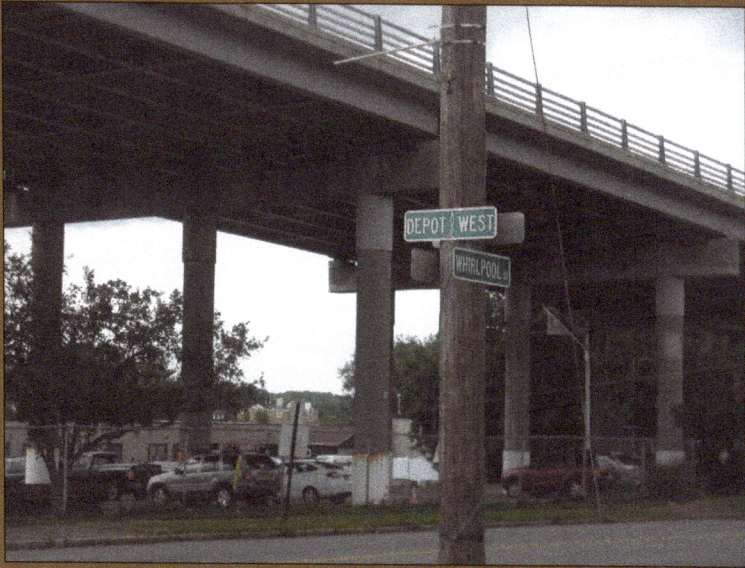

What's There Now?

Bellevue Mineral Spring was located west of Whirlpool Street at the end of Bath Avenue.

The Frontier House
2130 Whirlpool Street, Niagara Falls, NY

In 1850 John Vedder built this large three-story brick house on the extensive tract of land he owned in this area of Niagara Falls, which was then known as Bellevue. The Vedder property included the land that was later sold to the College and Seminary of Our Lady of the Angels (Niagara University).

John Vedder died in 1854, and his house was converted to the Globe Hotel in 1857. In this area of Bellevue, later called Suspension Bridge, there were many springs including the Bellevue Sulphur Spring, which was used for medicinal purposes. The Globe Hotel, which was re-named the Frontier House, was located on Spring Street; later the street name changed and the new address of the Frontier House was 2130 Whirlpool Street.

Down under the hill, right along the bank of the gorge, close by where the New York ends of the two great railway arches now stand, the early settlers located and called the place Bellevue. The rough street along which they built they called Spring Street, because adjacent to it were numerous springs sulphureous to the taste. Now the street is named Whirlpool Street.

Old Frontier House Once Boasted Of Sulphur Baths, Fine Falls View. By Marjorie F. Williams, City Historian, *Niagara Falls Gazette*, Tuesday, January 5, 1954.

In the 1880s Jacob A. Gutbrodt was the manager of the Frontier House, which at this early time was located on Spring Street, now known as Whirlpool Street. It was described as a handsome modern hotel with thirty guest rooms. The hotel was known for its sulphur baths and their healing abilities.

FRONTIER HOUSE, Suspension Bridge, N.Y. It is a handsome, modern building containing 30 large sleeping-rooms, excellent parlors, and all the modern conveniences. It is noted for its Sulphur Baths, which have been pronounced by medical men to be extremely beneficial in a large number of cutaneous and other diseases.

A complete record of Niagara Falls and vicinage by Thos. Holder 1892.

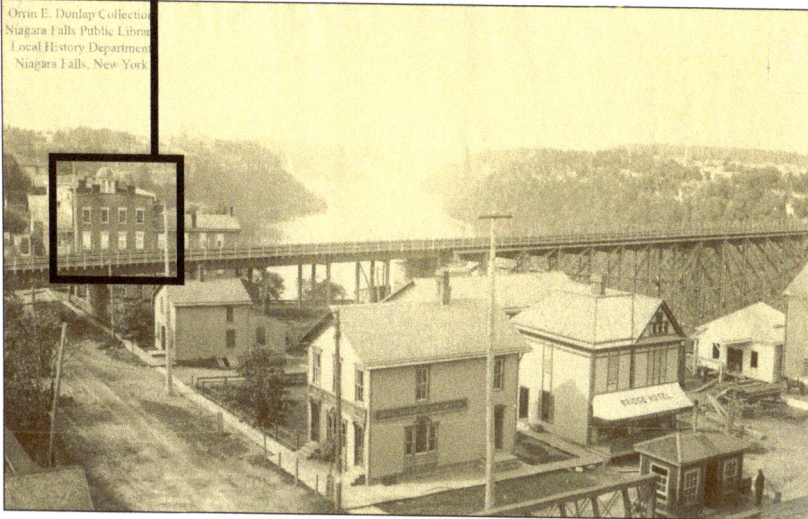

The Frontier House from an **1888** picture of Suspension Bridge facing South. Orrin E. Dunlap Collection, Niagara Falls Public Library, Local History Department, Niagara Falls, New York.

After 1902, the hotel name changed many times and no longer promoted the sulphur baths. A complete timeline of this historic building can be found on pages 147-148. This area of what was once Bellevue and Suspension Bridge had many industrial projects and the Suspension Bridge to Canada, the foundation of which is rumored to have cut off the flow of water to some of the springs, however the water from the springs continued to be used by the mineral spring hotels and local residents.

U.S. Customs House

Frontier House

Map of Niagara Falls (Suspension Bridge) with the Frontier House and the present-day Custom House Building noted, 1908.

What's There Now?

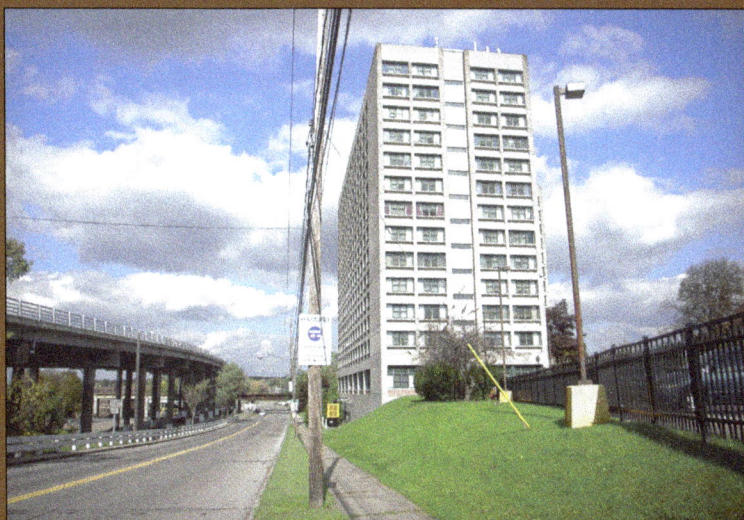

The Frontier House was located at the foot of Ontario Street on the upper bank of the Niagara River Gorge. Image is the corner of Whirlpool (was Spring) and Ontario streets, facing North.

The Monteagle Springs Sanitarium (Mineral Springs Hotel and Niagara Springs Sanatorium) Suspension Bridge, NY

The large and beautiful Monteagle Hotel had a long and colorful history. Constructed in 1848 of Niagara granite from the Niagara River gorge on over thirty acres of land, it had 150 rooms and a tower over 200 feet tall with an excellent view of the American and Canadian Falls, DeVeaux College, Ontario, Canada, and the nearby Suspension Bridge to Canada.

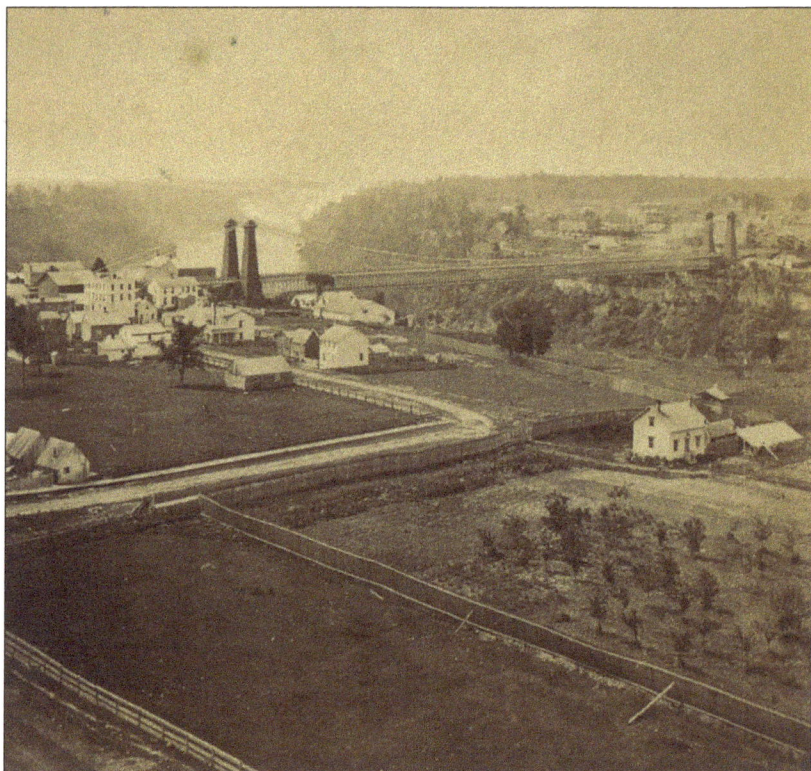

Distant view of Suspension Bridge from the Monteagle Tower. Stereoscopic view of the Falls, John P. Soul, photographer, #313.

The Monteagle Hotel was on a formation known as the Monteagle Ridge, which roughly follows the Niagara River northward. Niagara University is also on the Monteagle Ridge. The building had many uses and operated from 1855 to 1936, when it burned and was finally razed.

A legend about this area of Niagara Falls tells the story of a Native American couple who tragically threw themselves over the banks of the Niagara River. Their bodies were found at the mouth of the river still in an embrace. According to an article about the hotel, the previous owners of the land were the Seneca Nation of Indians who were forced to cede to the

British Crown in 1764, a strip of land two miles wide on each side of the Niagara River as reparation for the Devil's Hole Massacre in which eighty-one British soldiers were killed by Seneca warriors. The Niagara River reparation land was on the edge of the hotel grounds.

Early accounts record that there were several springs in the area that were used by the Native Americans and early settlers. A May 10, 1884, *Suspension Bridge Journal* article mentions that the Monteagle Springs Sanitarium was built on the grounds of a sanitarium used by Native Americans.

"It has about it large grounds, fronting it a beautiful grove and upon it Springs, wonderful traditions of whose healing powers have been handed down from the Indians who here established a rural Sanitarium centuries ago. It has been regarded as the most beautiful spot on the Niagara Frontier. The Mineral waters on the premises possess extraordinary curative virtues. Careful analysis shown that they contain Lime and Magnesia, in the form of sulphates and carbonated, Chloride of Sodium, Iron, Lithia and Potassium, all in combination with Sulphuretted Hydrogen and Carbonic Acid."

With the railroad stop at the back door, the Monteagle Hotel was in an excellent spot for travelers visiting Niagara Falls or traveling to Canada on the Suspension Bridge and for many years the hotel prospered. Shortly after opening in 1859, the Hotel following a health trend, introduced the healing powers of the Bellevue sulphur water that was nearby.

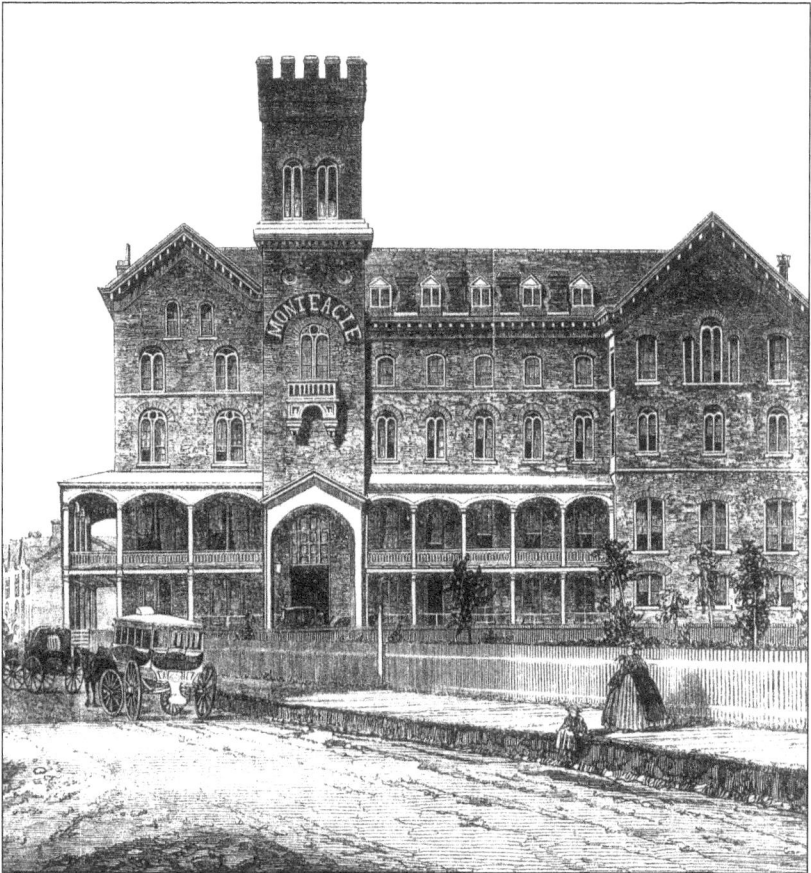

The Monteagle Hotel with its 200 foot tower. *The Illustrated London News*, vol. 43, no. 1218, p. 193. August 22, 1863.

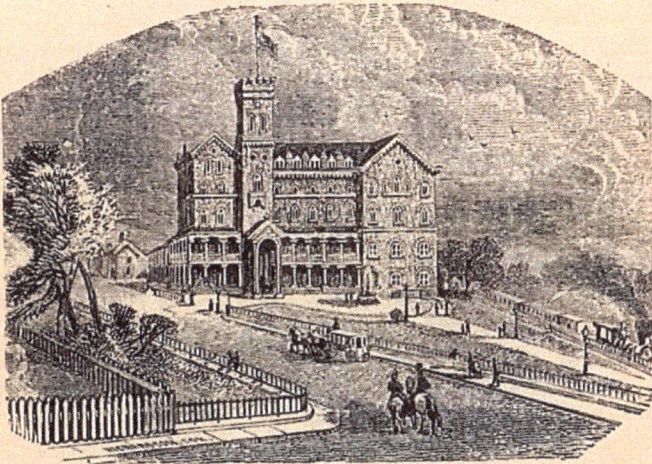

Monteagle House,

SUSPENSION BRIDGE, NIAGARA, N. Y.

This House is now open for the reception of its patrons and the traveling public, under an entire new management. Having been refitted and entirely renovated it commands the attention of parties visiting Niagara. The rooms command a fine, uninterrupted view of Niagara Falls, the two Suspension Bridges, Whirlpool, and Whirlpool Rapids. In connection with the house are Mineral Sulpher Springs and Baths, making it desirable for those requiring tonic and cutaneous treatment.

Free Omnibus to and from all trains.

TERMS, $3.00 per day.

Special inducements to parties remaining any length of time. Parties intending to stop at the Monteagle, should have their baggage checked to Suspension Bridge.

ALEXANDER & TERRILL, Proprietors.

15

Advertisement for the Monteagle House. For a short time (1875–1876), Alexander & Terrill operated the Hotel as the Monteagle House, utilizing the mineral sulphur springs.

Home for the Elderly

The hotel changed ownership several times and went into foreclosure in 1876. The next reported use was by an Alexian Brother by the name of Brother Paul for use as a home for aging clerics. Although reported in the *Niagara Falls Gazette* several times, it is not clear if Brother Paul opened his home for the elderly. The archives of the Order do not have records of the facility but do indicate that Brother Paul was attempting to open an Alexian Brothers institution in New York in 1879–1880.

The Index says the purchasers of the Monteagle Hotel property are the Alexian Brothers, and that the place is to be converted into a home for clergymen who have grown old and infirm in the work of the ministry. Dec. 3, 1879

Stone is being quarried near the Seminary of Our Lady of Angels to be used in building a stone wall around the old Monteagle Hotel, which is being converted into a home for infirm and aged Catholic clergy. March 24, 1880

Niagara Falls Gazette, March 24, 1880, and December 3, 1879. Local articles indicating that Brother Paul was involved in establishing a home for elderly clergymen.

The Alexian Brothers

A Catholic affiliated Christian health charity founded in the twelfth century in Europe. Now a large progressive health organization with facilities in the United States, the Philippines, Hungary, Great Britain, Ireland, Germany, and Belgium. Most of their service is to the poor, elderly people with mental health issues, AIDS patients, and other marginalized groups.

"An Alexian Brother by the name of Brother Paul (Paulus) Pollig (secular name Mathias Pollig) ran afoul of his superiors in Aachen, Germany in the 1870s. Brother Paul arrived in America from Aachen in 1866, and was an important part of the expansion of the ministry here. Since we know that Paul was determined to establish an Alexian institution in America outside of the formal congregation, and we know that he received encouragement in New York, it is possible that Paul started something in Niagara Falls. We do not know what he was doing during the period between November 1878 and August of 1879."

Research Library Alexian Brothers, 2011

Monteagle Springs Sanitarium

In 1884, with much local publicity, Dr. Crumb converted the former Monteagle Hotel to The Monteagle Springs Sanitarium, a full treatment spring resort with Turkish, Russian, and medicated vapor baths, thermal medicated baths, electro medicated baths, vacuum cure massage, and the Swedish Movement Cure.[1]

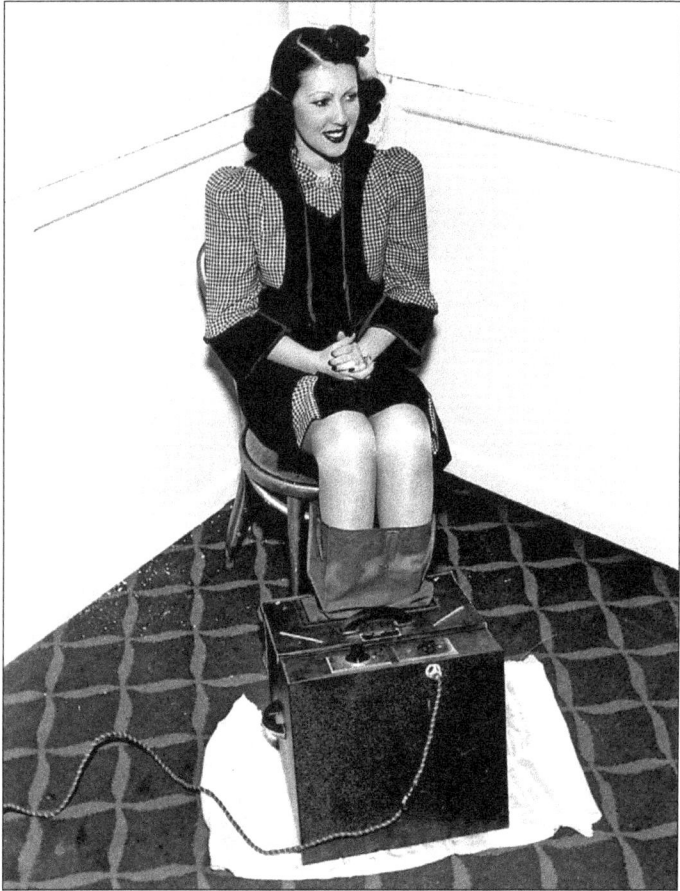

Electric Medicated Vapor Bath. Designed to relive tired muscles, stimulate circulation and reduce inflammation, one of the hotel's treatments. Museum of disABILITY History archives.

The May 10, 1884, *Suspension Bridge Journal* had a full-page advertisement on the opening of the Monteagle Springs Sanitarium. *The Medina Register*, May 22, 1884, reported that the renovated Monteagle at Suspension Bridge was open to the public, and the sanitarium department would open in thirty days.

Dr. Crumb graduated from the College of Physicians & Surgeons in Buffalo in 1882 and Bennett College of Eclectic Medicine & Surgery in Chicago, 1884. He was an entrepreneur in the healing business with documentation showing that he was an agent for Athol Mineral Spring water and the facilities at the Athol House, Hamburg, NY. He also was an inventor of several medicines including Crumb's Hard Rubber Pocket Inhaler, Crumb's Carbonic Ointment, and Crumb's Compound Pills. He managed a small sanitarium in Buffalo before moving with his son to Niagara Falls.

Dr. Crumb's pocket inhaler.

Warner's Safe Nervine, Rochester, NY. Dr. Crumb claimed it cured his depression.

CRUMB'S COMPOUND PILLS
---OF---
Butternut and May-Apple.

-----HAVE-------NOT-----THEIR------EQUAL - ---

For Purifying the Blood and acting powerfully,
yet soothing, on the Liver, Stomach, Kidneys
and Bowels, giving Tone, Energy, and Vigor
to the whole system. They are wonderfully
efficacious in Billions Attacks, Constipation,
and in connection with Crumb's Carbolic
Ointment, for Piles.

Price per bottle, 15 cents.   Sold by all druggists.
Manufactured by   CRUMB & CO.
9dyi   Buffalo, N.Y.

Dr. Crumb's compound pills.

As Dr. Crumb was interviewed for an article about the
new Monteagle Springs Sanitarium, he recounted his struggle
with severe depression and mentioned that he opened the
Sanitarium in the hopes that he could help others with similar
conditions. He was a proponent of Warner's Safe Cure
Nervine, a patent medicine that he claimed released him from
his depression.

The Monteagle Springs Sanitarium operated for just over a
year when Dr. Crumb retired.

TREATMENT OF DISTANT PATIENTS

An extensive correspondence is carried on in all parts of the United States, Canada and elsewhere. Sufferers from chronic diseases who are unable to visit the Sanitarium, receive treatment by mail. Upon receipt of the name and address, a list of questions is sent, full and explicit answers to which enable the Doctor to form a correct diagnosis of each case. Asthma, Catarrh, Consumption, Paralysis, and other diseases hitherto regarded as incurable, are treated with success unparalleled in the medical history of the world. The fees are within the reach of all, and patients at home and abroad receive the kindest consideration and sympathy. Correspondence is cordially solicited. Send stamp for pamphlet.

Address,

DR. W. R. CRUMB,

Monteagle Springs, Suspension Bridge, NY.

Dr. W. R. Crumb's mail-order medical business.

SANITARIUM,

Suspension Bridge, N. Y.

Is Now Open!

To Travellers, Tourists, Rest - Seekers and Permanent Guests.

———o———

The Monteagle Springs Sanitarium presents unsurpassed attractions for Travellers, Tourists, Rest Seekers and Permanent Guests. The spacious and beautiful edifice at Suspension Bridge formerly known as the Monteagle Hotel, has been thoroughly refitted and re-opened for that purpose.

No other health resort in the country combines greater advantages of pure and bracing air, beauty of situation and accessibility of health-giving waters.

The building itself surpasses in beauty and commodiousness any similar institution in the world. It has about it large grounds, fronting it a beautiful grove and upon it Springs, wonderful traditions of whose healing powers have been handed down from the Indians who here established a rural Sanitarium centuries ago. It has long been regarded as the most beautiful spot on the Niagara Frontier.

One of the advantages of this Sanitarium is that it is located at a railroad center and is remarkably convenient of access from all parts of the country. Here is the terminus of the New York Central, Erie, West Shore, Rome, Watertown and Ogdensburgh, Lehigh Valley, Grand Trunk and Michigan Central Railroads. Three of them leave passengers on the Sanitarium landing and the depots of the others are within three minutes walk.

Free Omnibus connects with every train. Terms will be liberal with special rates to permanent boarders. Persons desiring rooms for the season will do well to communicate early. For further particulars address

DR. W. R. CRUMB,

Monteagle Springs, Suspension Bridge, N. Y.

Advertising for the opening of the Monteagle Springs Sanitarium, 1884. *Suspension Bridge Journal*, May 10, 1884.

The Mineral Springs Hotel

The Hotel was turned over to John B. Manning (former Mayor of Buffalo), who opened the Mineral Springs Hotel. On April 8, 1885, a *Niagara Falls Gazette* article mentions that the building will be both a hotel and a sanitarium. "On the grounds is a white sulphur spring, the water of which contains rare medicinal and curative qualities. The medical department will be under the charge and supervision of one of the most skillful and capable physicians in the country, who will be assisted by a full staff of the best specialists. The hotel and sanitarium will be first-class in all its appointments. Connected with the sanitarium will be Mineral, Turkish, Russian, Hot air, Sitz plunge and Electro-Thermal baths, Massage, and the Swedish movement cure will also be introduced." [2]

A large park, Whirlpool Rapids Park, was opened by the hotel in 1886; it stretched from the hotel on Lewiston Road to the banks of the Niagara River. On the grounds were white sulphur, lithia, and crystal springs. There was a double elevator and a staircase descending to a viewing platform that overlooked the rapids.

Swedish Movement Cure
The Swedish Movements are a series of systematic exercise therapeutically applied to the human body. One of the many treatments offered by the Mineral Spring Hotel.

The Niagara Springs Sanatorium

NIAGARA SPRINGS SANATORIUM
SUSPENSION BRIDGE, N.Y.
(OPEN ALL THE YEAR)

For the treatment of all chronic diseases, such as Rheumatism, Sciatica, Gout, Dyspepsia, Liver and Kidney Diseases, Heart and Lung Diseases, Nervous Diseases, Spinal Deformities, Plica and all diseases of the skin.

Diseases are treated according to methods adopted in Edinburgh, London and Germany.

Diseases peculiar to women are treated by a specialist of wide experience.

THE BATHING DEPARTMENT

Is completed in all particulars and under direct medical supervision. The only Turkish, Russian, Medicinal and Electrical Baths administered in Niagara Falls or the vicinity. Street cars come from Niagara Falls to the Sanitorium every 15 minutes.

Gentleman's Hours

Monday, Wednesday, Thursday, Saturday	8am to 6pm
Thursday and Friday Afternoons	2-6
Wednesday and Saturday Evenings	6-9
Saturday Morning	7-12

Ladies Hours

Tuesday and Friday	8am-1pm

Season Tickets, entitling to 10 Turkish, Russian or Turco-Russian Baths for $15.00

Niagara Springs Sanatorium advertising. *Suspension Bridge Journal,* December 31, 1887.

In 1887, Drs. Bell and Thompson opened the Niagara Springs Sanatorium. The Niagara Springs Sanatorium claimed to cure Rheumatism, liver and kidney diseases, nervous diseases, spinal deformations, piles, and diseases of the skin.[3]

The Monteagle Lithia Spring

The Monteagle Springs Hotel at Suspension Bridge, (Niagara Falls) NY, also utilized in the treatments a spring that contained lithium. Lithium was discovered as a health cure in the early nineteenth century and there is evidence that lithia springs were previously used by Native Americans as a health aid.

Lithium is a mineral salt substance that has been used to treat alcoholism, opium addiction, and in a refined form is presently used to treat mood disorders (bipolar disorder).

The lithia springs water from Lithia Springs, Georgia, lists benefits to the following problems: Attention Deficit Disorder, Bi-polar, Depression, Post-partum Depression, Alzheimer's disease, and Sleep disorders.[4]

One of the first drinks with lithium was Bib-Label Lithiated lemon-lime soda. "You Like it, it Likes You!" It was later renamed 7up. The lithium was eventually removed. Mountain Dew soda also started out as a lithiated drink.

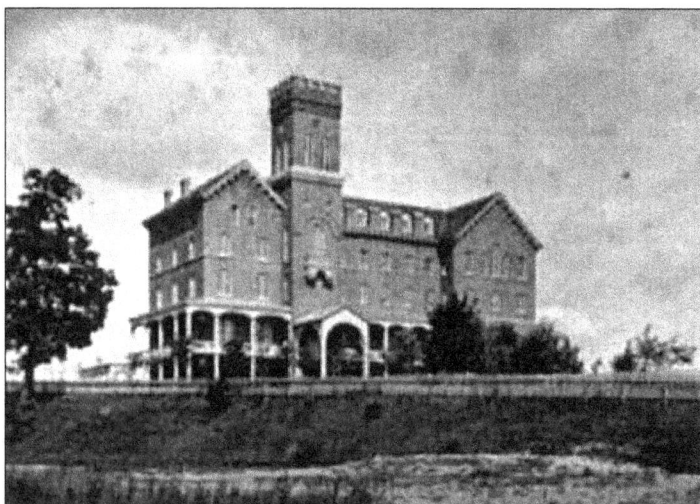

Monteagle Springs Hotel, which had a Lithia Spring on the property.

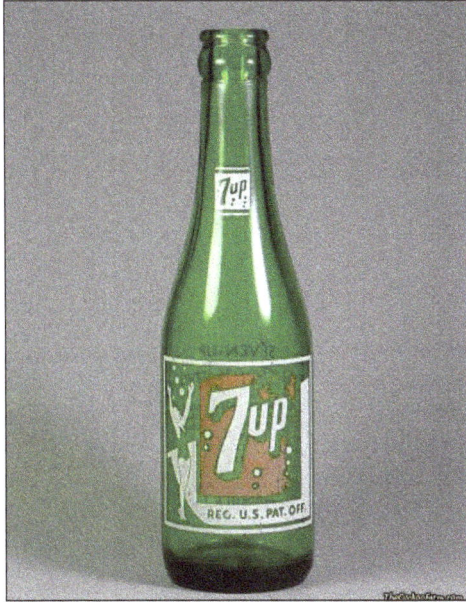

One of the first Lithium drinks was 7up.

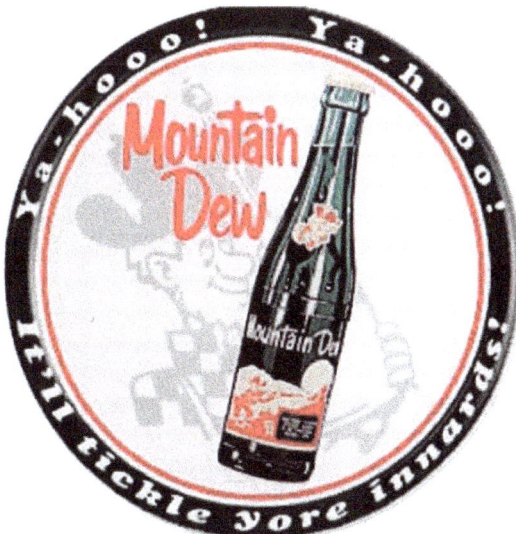

Mountain Dew started as a Lithium Drink.

No Longer a Hotel

In 1888, the fancy Monteagle Hotel, which utilized the nearby Mineral Springs to function as a health facility for over twenty-nine years, was purchased from John B. Manning by Willis and Burt Van Horn, Niagara County farmers, for use as cold storage for their farm products.

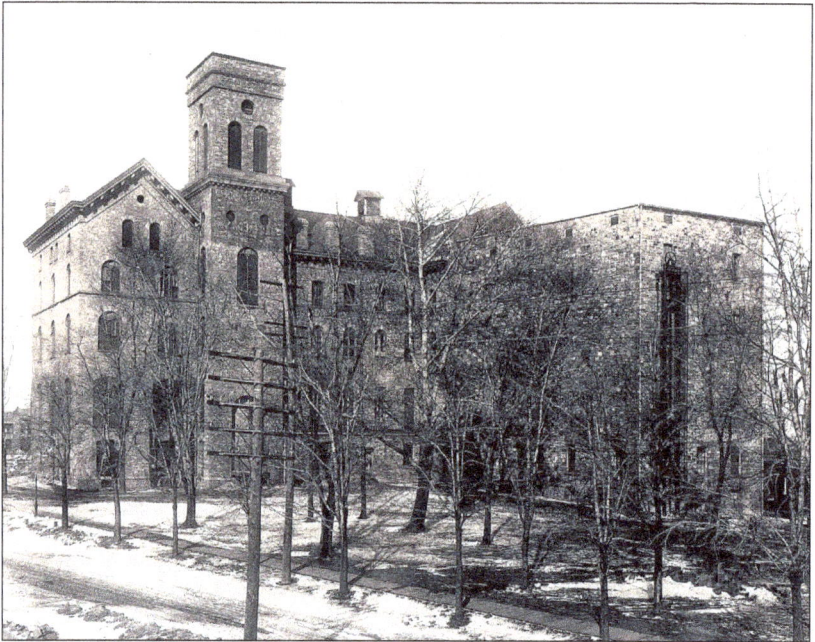

No longer a hotel, the Monteagle functioned as a cold storage building (Believed to be the 1930s).

From 1888 until the 1930s, it was used by a variety of businesses such as a cold storage, a coal company, and an icehouse.

In 1936, while being readied for demolition, a fire burned what remained of the once proud Monteagle Hotel.

The Monteagle Hotel burns to the ground in 1937.

The Monteagle House Timeline

1848-54: Built
1855-1878: Operated as hotel
1879-1880: Alexian Brothers Home for the Elderly
1884-1888: Sanitarium
1888: Cold Storage: VanHorn purchased hotel and converted it Suspension
Bridge Cold Storage Warehouse Co. Final owners ran the Cataract
Ice Company at the former hotel.
1937: Fire
1937: Building razed

An extensive timetable of the Monteagle House is found on pages 149–151.

Believed to be Pump House for
the Monteagle's spring water.

Mont Eagle Hotel

Niagara Falls, 1908, with the Monteagle Hotel and the Hotel Mineral
Water Pump House indicated.

What's there now?

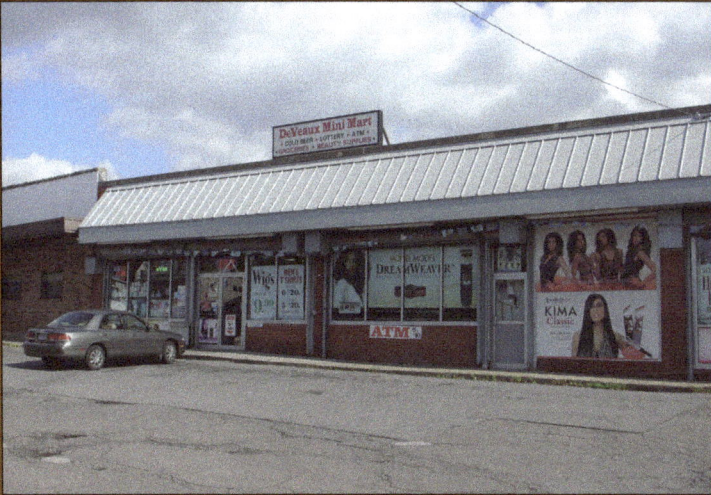

DeVeaux MiniMart, 2649 Main Street, Niagara Falls, New York. On grounds of former Monteagle Hotel.

CHAPTER 2

Alternative Medicine Sanitariums

Dr. Hodge's Sanitarium
Niagara Falls, NY, 1897–1900

I n 1897, Dr. William H. Hodge of Niagara Falls formed a stock company and raised $100,000 to open a health facility. Dr. Hodge then purchased the former Gaskill House at 424 Pine Ave, Niagara Falls, NY, in what is now known as the Historical Park Place District, and converted the facility to Dr. Hodge's Sanitarium with both Dr. William Hodge and his brother, John Hodge, as practitioners. The Board of Directors were Charles S. Marley of Detroit and John W. Hodge and Allan H. Hardwick of Niagara Falls.[1,2]

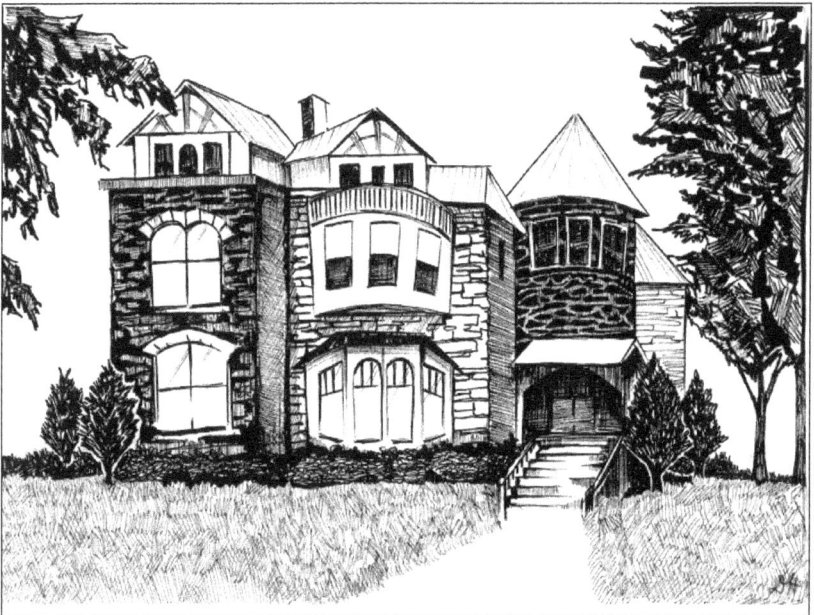

Dr. Hodge's Sanitarium. 424 Pine Avenue, Niagara Falls, NY. This drawing, by Danielle Herrmann, is from a poor-quality image in newspaper files.

The Dr. Hodge Sanitarium.

Niagara Falls will soon have one of the finest sanitariums in the country. A company with a capital of $100,000, at the head of which are the Drs. Hodge, will erect a large and handsome structure Dr. W. H. Hodge will be in charge of the institution. The building will be of the Old Colonial style, elaborately furnished, with all modern improvements that taste and ingenuity can devise. We wish Drs. Hodge abundant success in their commendable enterprise.

Medical ERA. Jan-Dec 1898, Vol. XVL

Dr. Hodge's Sanitarium had a capacity of fifty beds. This was a homeopathic treatment hospital and both brothers were homeopathic physicians.

Both William Hodge and his brother John were residents of Niagara County, NY. They grew up on a farm in Cambria, NY. Their father was James Hodge, a successful farmer, and their mother was Catherine. On June 6, 1898, William Hodge married Miss Clara Virginia Eaton of Lockport, NY, and moved with his new wife to the Sanitarium at 424 Pine Ave., Niagara Falls, NY. Dr. William H. Hodge and his brother Dr. John W. Hodge were in practice together with their offices at the Sanitarium; however, William H. Hodge is listed as the executive director of the Sanitarium. William Hodge, MD, and his brother John Hodge, MD, also retained offices at the Gluck building in Niagara Falls.[1]

In 1910, William Hodge was President of the New York State Homeopathic Society.

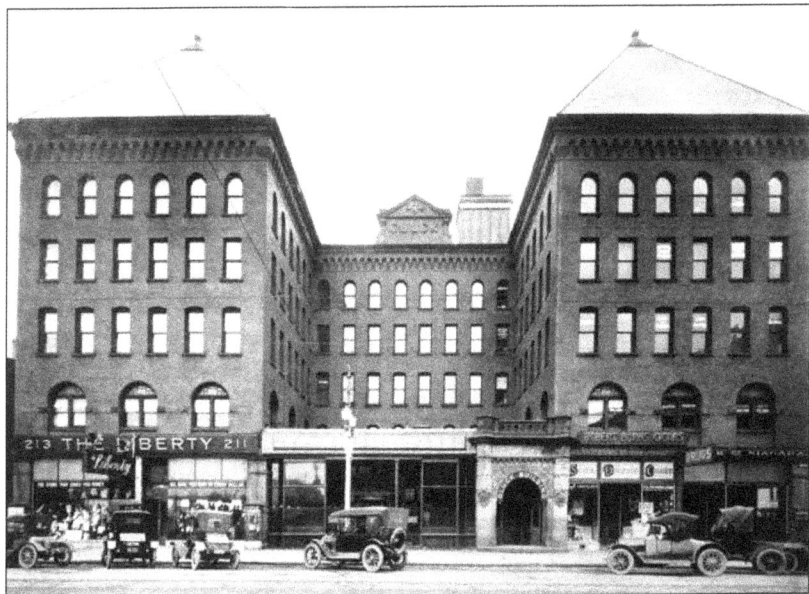

Gluck building in Niagara Falls. Both William Hodge, MD, and his brother John Hodge, MD, had offices in the building.

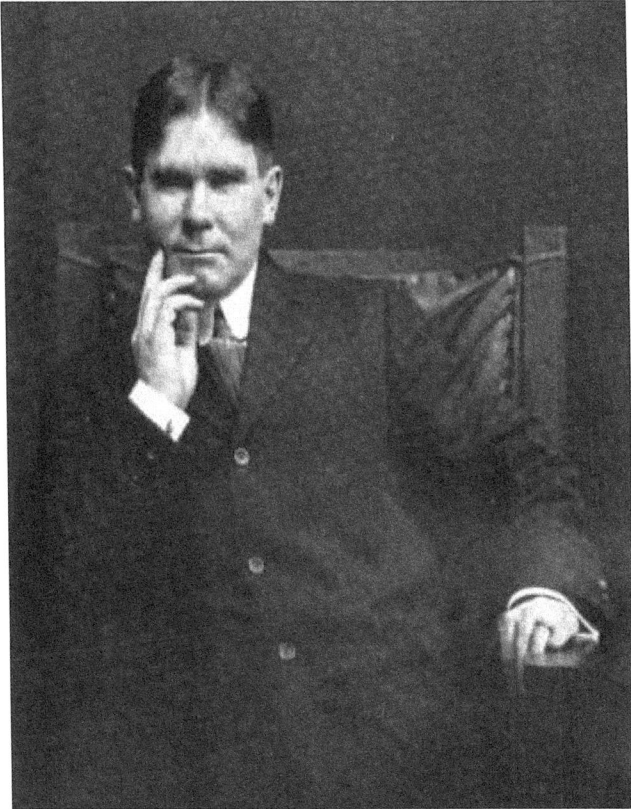

Dr. William H. Hodge. Recently elected president of the
New York State Homeopathic Society. *Niagara Falls
Gazette*, Feb. 16, 1910.

Dr. John W. Hodge was a strong supporter of homeopathic medicine, and the following is a famous quote of his that is used extensively in current writings and books about alternative medicine.

> " The medical monopoly or medical trust, euphemistically called the American Medical Association, is not merely the meanest monopoly ever organized, but the most arrogant, dangerous and despotic organization which ever managed a free people in this or any other age. Any and all methods of healing the sick by means of safe, simple and natural remedies are sure to be assailed and denounced by the arrogant leaders of the AMA doctors' trust as fakes, frauds and humbugs. Every practitioner of the healing art who does not ally himself with the medical trust is denounced as a 'dangerous quack' and impostor by the predatory trust doctors. Every sanitarian who attempts to restore the sick to a state of health by natural means without resort to the knife or poisonous drugs, disease imparting serums, deadly toxins or vaccines, is at once pounced upon by these medical tyrants and fanatics, bitterly denounced, vilified and persecuted to the fullest extent."[3]

The historic Gaskill Mansion was built in 1887 by Col. Charles B. Gaskill. Besides its use as a sanitarium, it was also a private home and functioned (on and off) as medical offices. In 1969 the building was demolished, and a new medical arts building was constructed and is now on the site.

What's there now?

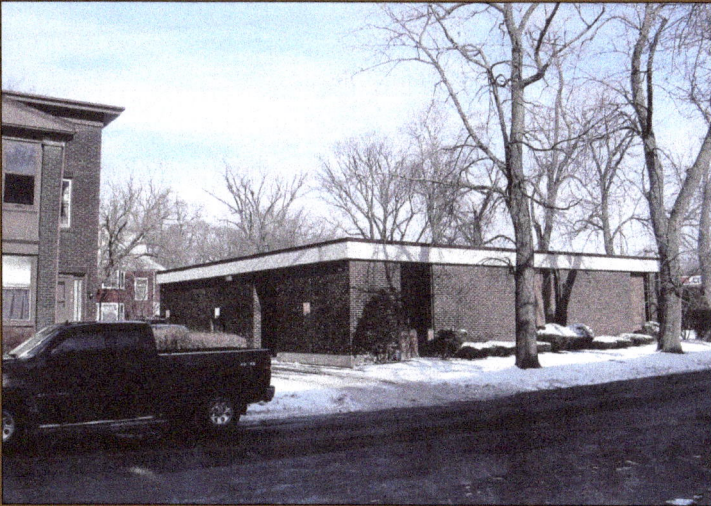

Site of the former Gaskill House and Dr. Hodge's Sanitarium, 424 Pine Avenue (now 416 Pine and 700 Park Place), Niagara Falls, NY. The former Gaskill Mansion and Hodges Sanitarium was removed in 1969 and replaced in 1971 with this Medical Arts Building.

The Electro-Magnetic Sanitarium
1901

On May 22, 1901, the *Daily Cataract Journal* reported that the Kingsley Mansion was leased to Professor Benard of Buffalo and was open for business as the Electro-Magnetic Sanitarium. The Sanitarium was located in a large house formerly owned by John C. Lammerts on the corner of Ferry and 6th streets, Niagara Falls, NY.

The medical director of the Electro-Magnetic Sanitarium was Dr. Kennedy who was also the president of the National Medical Institute and Hospital of Buffalo, NY. Professor B. B. Benard who was associated with the Electro-Magnetic Institute, Buffalo, was the director of the Niagara Falls Sanitarium. Professor Benard used his extraordinary diagnostic skills to market the sanitarium and would offer the service at no cost. The promotional material for the Electro-Magnetic listed a staff of physicians, surgeons, osteopaths, and Magnetic and Mental Healers. Also employed was the X-ray and "Electro-Therapeutics" for the caring of all chronic nervous and mental disorders.[4,5,6,7]

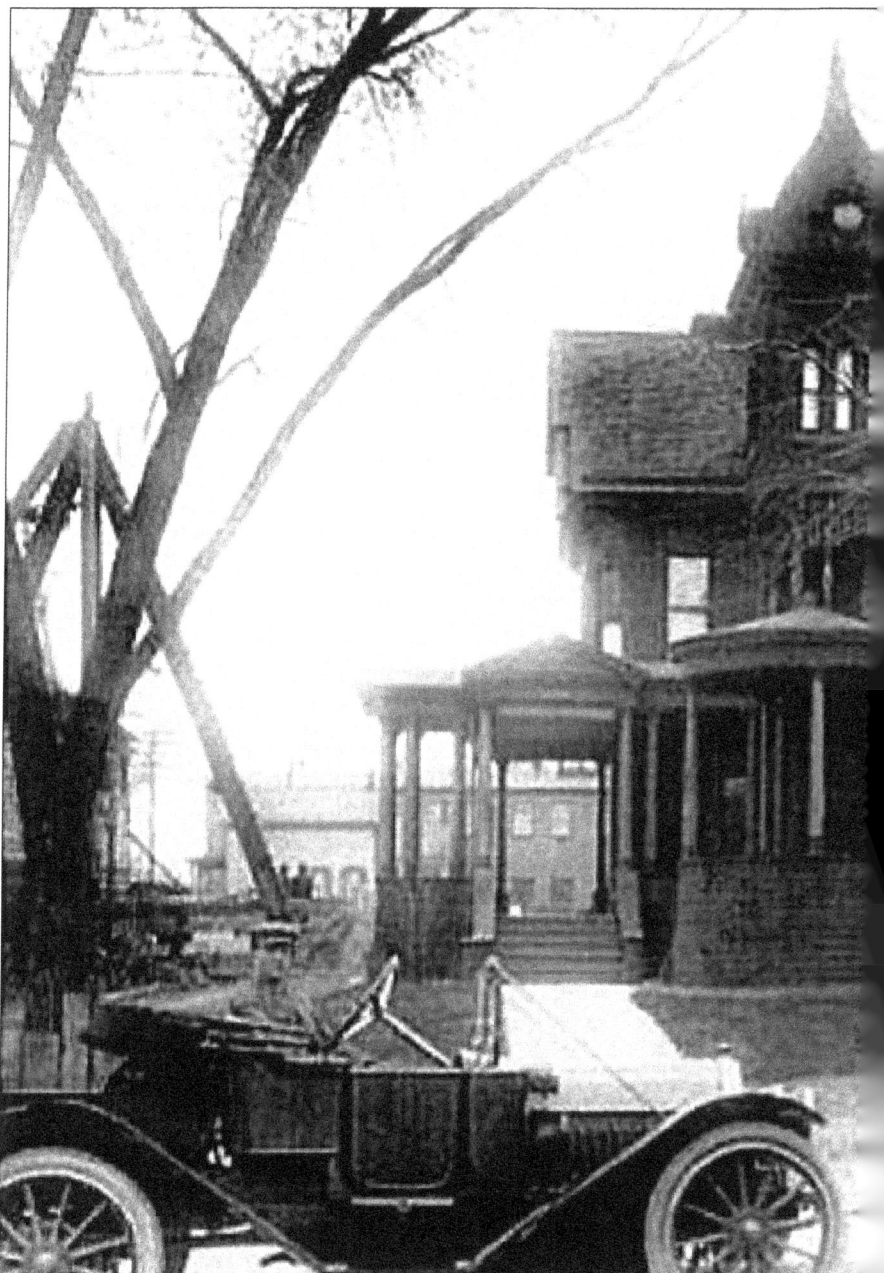

The Electro-Magnetic Sanitarium of Niagara Falls, corner of Ferry and 6th Streets.

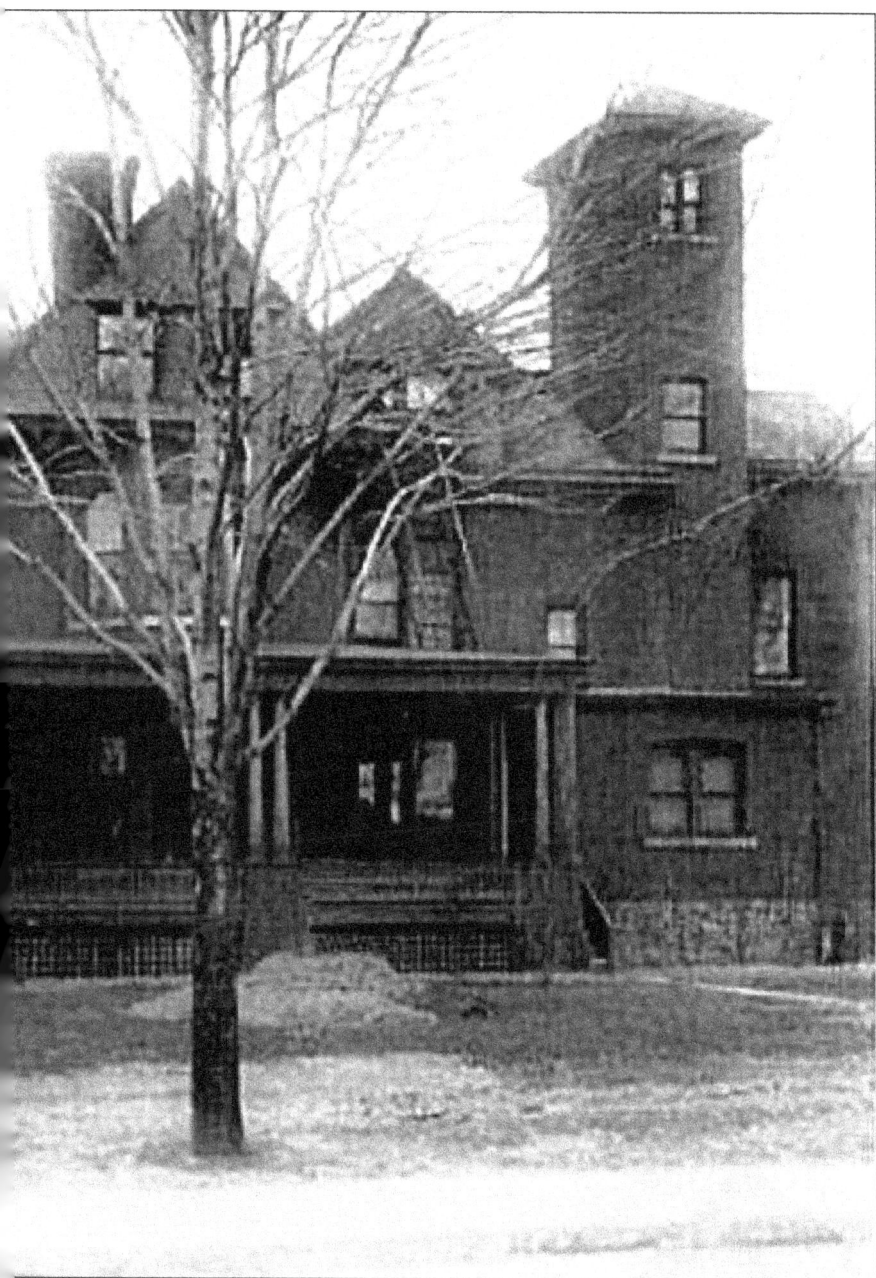

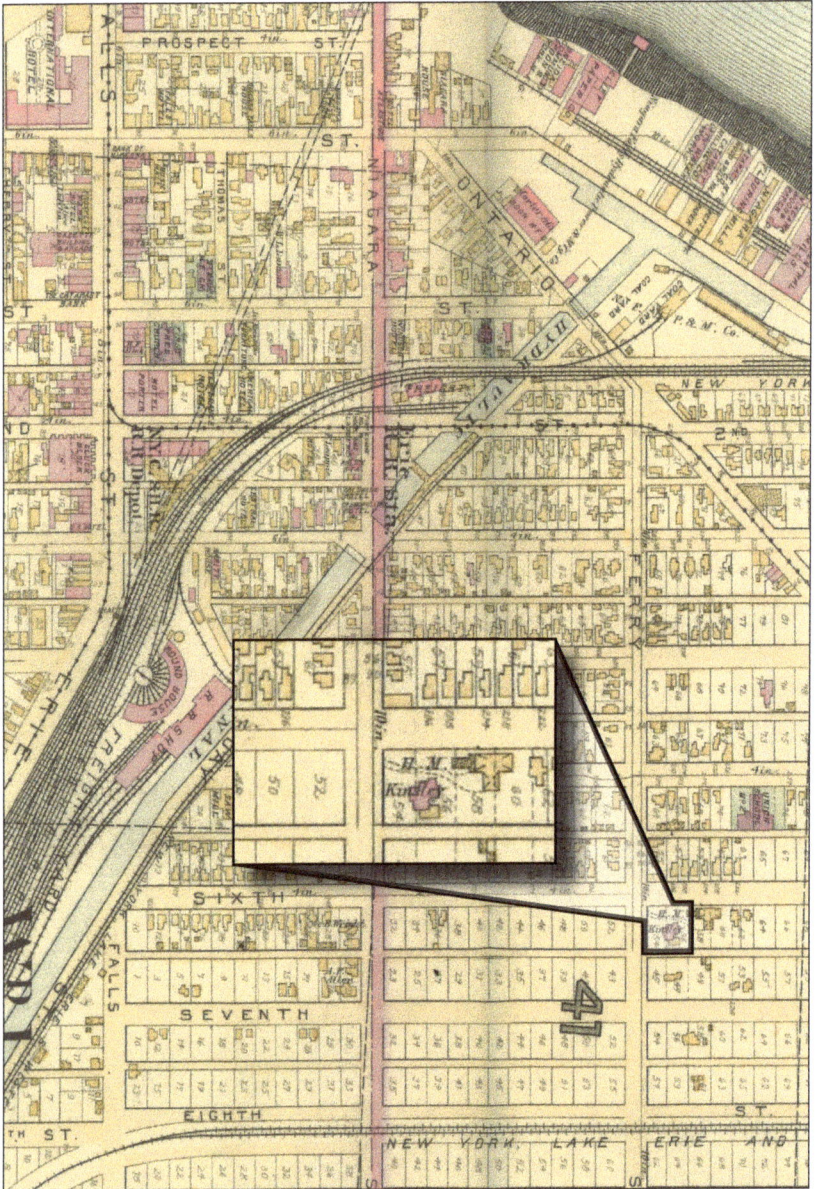

Site of the Electro-Magnetic Sanitarium in the former Kingsley Mansion - Ferry and 6th streets, Niagara Falls, NY. Ward Maps, G.M. Hopkins & Co., 1893.

PROF BENARD WILL BE THERE

Next Tuesday, October 28th, Prof. Benard will devote one entire day at 222 Third Street in diagnosing disease. He tells you the nature and symptoms of your disease and all about your ailments without asking a single question. Examinations and consultations free. One day only. Hours 10 a.m. until 5 p.m.

The director of the Electro-Magnetic Sanitarium, Professor Benard, had unique diagnostic skills. *Niagara Falls Gazette:* October 25, 1902.

The Electro-Magnetic Institute closed in 1906 and Mount St. Mary's Hospital was started in the large mansion in 1907. It was known as "The Little House on the Corner." Later, the new Mount St. Mary's Hospital was built on the mansion grounds.

What's there now?

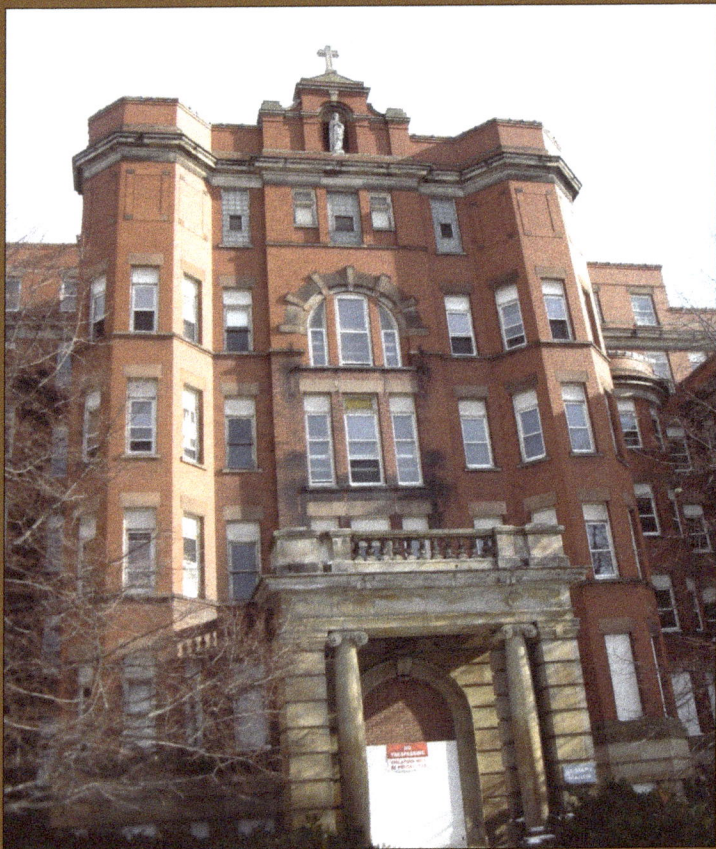

Location of the Electro-Magnetic Sanitarium. The former Mount St. Mary's Hospital and Nursing Home, corner of Ferry and 6th streets, Niagara Falls, NY. The Hospital moved in 1965 to Lewiston, NY.

CHAPTER 3

Hotel Based
Water Treatments

Bath (Green) Island Bath Houses
Niagara Falls, NY

Bath Island had a number of bath houses built in the 1830s located along the western side of the island. In 1895 the name was changed from Bath Island to Green Island after Andrew H. Green, a Niagara Reservation Commissioner.

The bath houses channeled the river currents of the fast-moving Niagara River and used this power to provide a forceful healthy jet stream of water to clients. They offered both warm and cold baths.

> Bath Island was, by reason of the world-famed current baths, the first place erected where one could safely dip oneself in the running waters of Niagara."

Official Guide: Niagara Falls – River Frontier Peter A. Porter, 1901

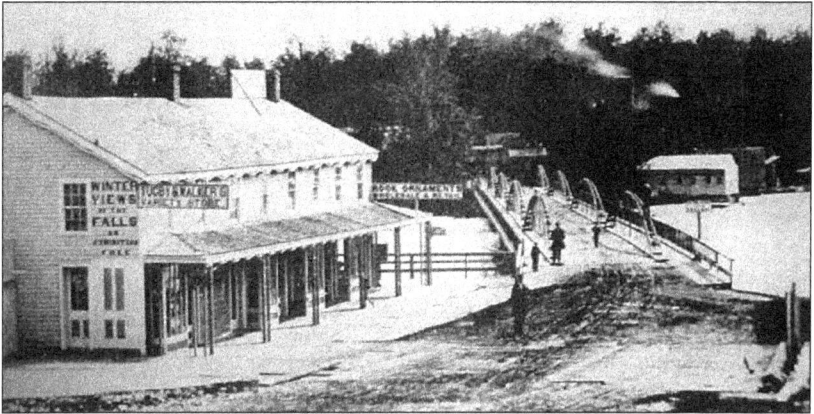

This is the bridge to Bath Island. The buildings to the right were the Bath Houses. Tugby's store is to the left. 1866 Photograph. *Buffalo Courier Express* 6/20/1976.

The island was once called Bath Island for the bathhouse, which opened here in 1821. This establishment offered, "showering baths, as well as warm and cold baths from the rushing waters of the rapids." The baths became world-famous, and many people believed the limestone minerals in the water would cure their physical ailments. Bath Island was renamed Green Island in the 1880's in honor of Andrew H. Green, a president and a member of the Board of Commissioners of the State Reservation at Niagara."[1]

Bath Island is largely man-made with stone and coal cinders on a rock base and six inches of loam. The records indicate a bath house on the Island with Niagara current, hot and cold, and plunge baths. The baths were noted for keeping long hours as they were open until 11PM. In 1849, they were operated by a Mr. M. L. Fox and described as "kept in the best order."[1, 2]

Bath Island was cleaned up in the 1880s by the Park Commission and the mills and bath houses were removed.

The rough industrial and tourist area around the falls was seized by New York State with the use of eminent domain. Over 150 buildings were renovated or relocated. A 139- acre park, The Niagara Reservation, designed around the recommendations of Frederick Law Olmstead was created in 1885 with the intent to restore the natural beauty of the site.

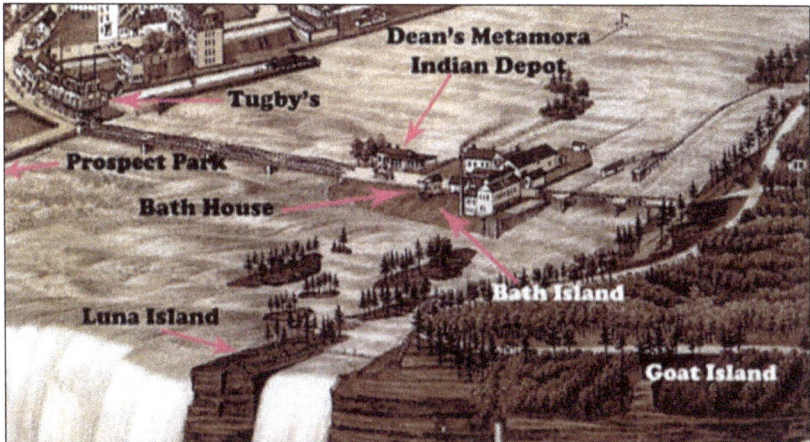

Bath island 1882 with the bathhouse noted.[3]

What's there now?

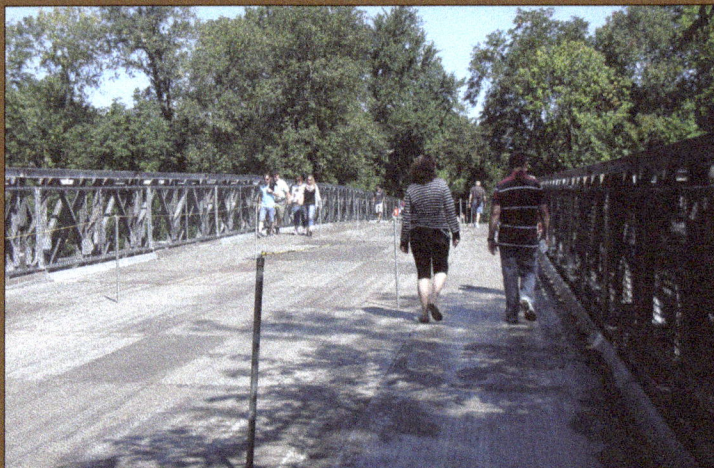

Bridge to Green (Bath) Island from Goat Island.

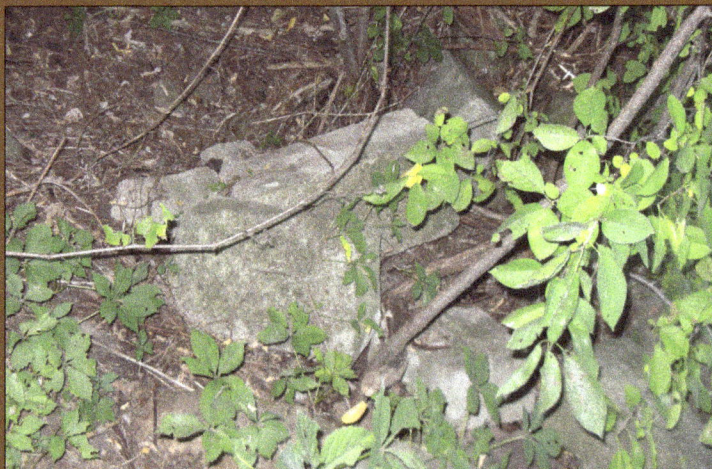

Once you get off the bridge and mowed lawn area, there is evidence of the Island's former history. Building materials and cut stone are found along the edge of the water. Bath Island, 2013.

The Cataract House Hotel

This hotel and baths utilized the fast-moving currents of the Niagara River to offer their clients a healthful, vigorous bath often with curative claims. The baths operated from the 1820s until the Niagara Commission removed most of the commercial businesses and restored the Falls and Niagara River area in the 1880s.

The Cataract House Hotel was located on the bank of the upper Niagara River near the bridge that crossed to Bath Island (Green Island).

The expanded Cataract House Hotel was built in 1825 on the Niagara River just above Niagara Falls. The Cataract House Hotel utilized the roaring current from the Niagara River to provide a strong bathing experience to its guests. In the building was an open mill race that provided a vigorous current bath as it flowed through the basement area into the bathing basins. A Cataract House timeline is found on page 153-154.

"Bathing in running water was years ago regarded as highly beneficial to cases of nervous disorders. Such baths are held to be of value in nervous disorders, for imagination plays a large part in the cure of many such cases."

The Buffalo Express, Nov. 12, 1900.

" There is a great and uncommon luxury in the lower regions of this hotel: a couple of strong-current baths; that is to say, a small stream is diverted from the troubled rapids that boil past the house at lightning-speed towards the falls and is led through a hole in the wall into two baths that resemble large troughs about twelve feet long, five feet broad, and two and a half feet deep, in which the bather disports himself, approaching as near as possible to the aperture about a yard from the ground, through which the torrent hurls itself with a velocity that carries it three or four feet before it falls to the bottom of the bath, afterwards disappearing more mildly through a grating at the other end. Immersion in this for a few minutes in hot weather is exceedingly grateful and refreshing."

Reminiscences of America in 1869
Alex Rivington, Harris (English writer on America)

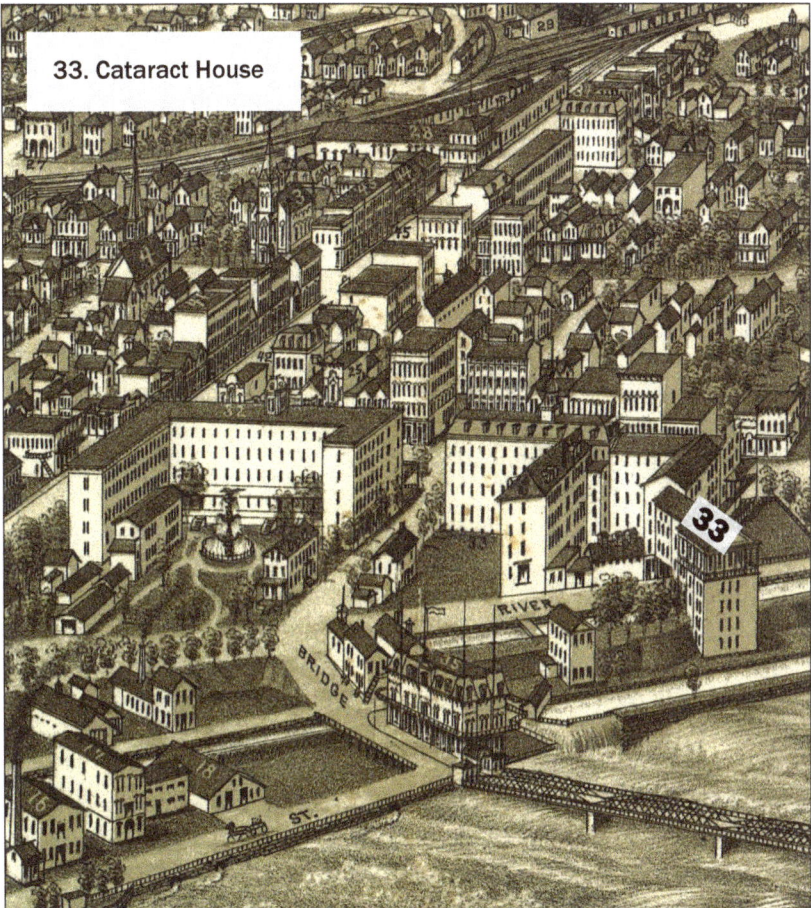

Niagara Falls, NY, 1882. The bridge to Bath Island (Green Island), local hotels, and the image of the Cataract House on the Niagara Rapids.[4]

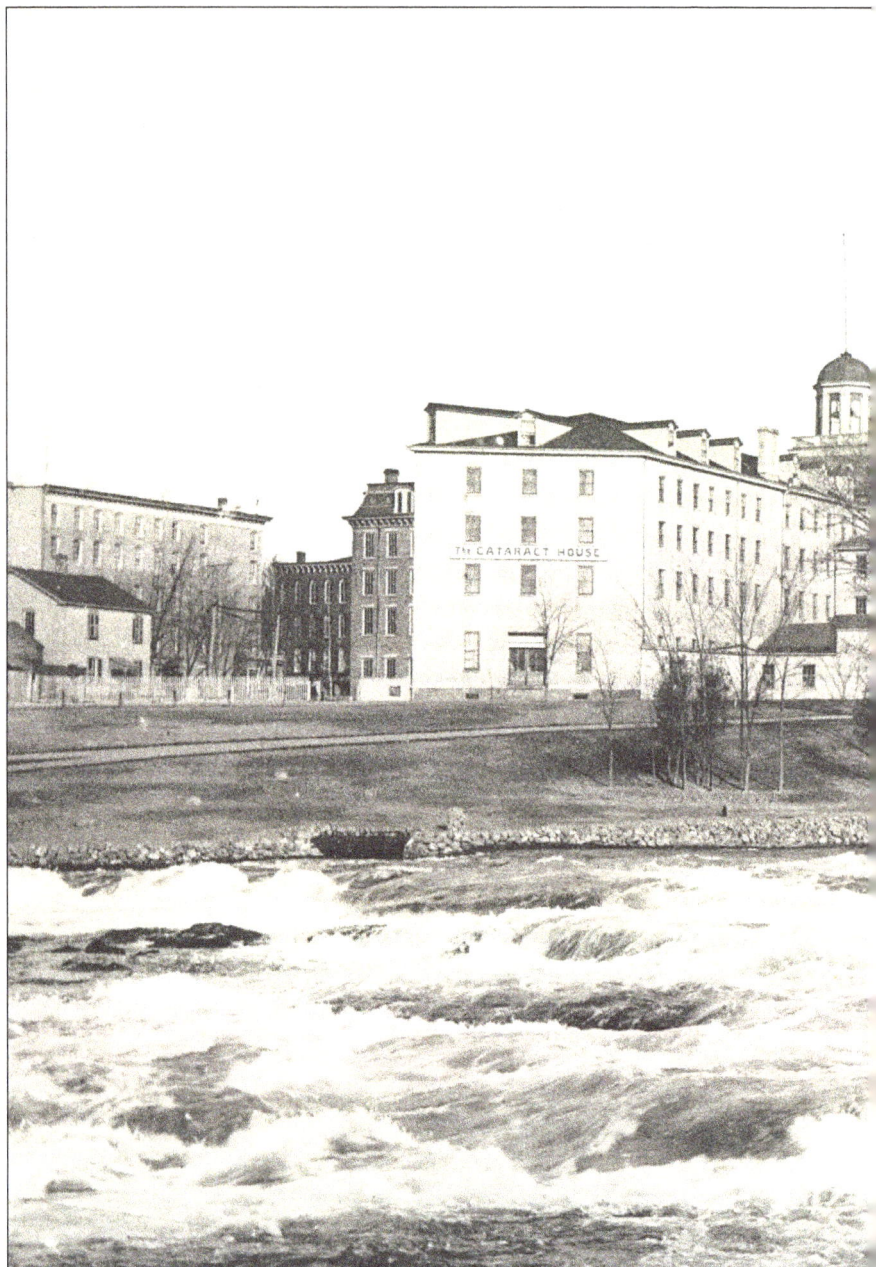

The first building on the site was the Eagle Tavern, which was rebuilt and became the Cataract House in 1825.

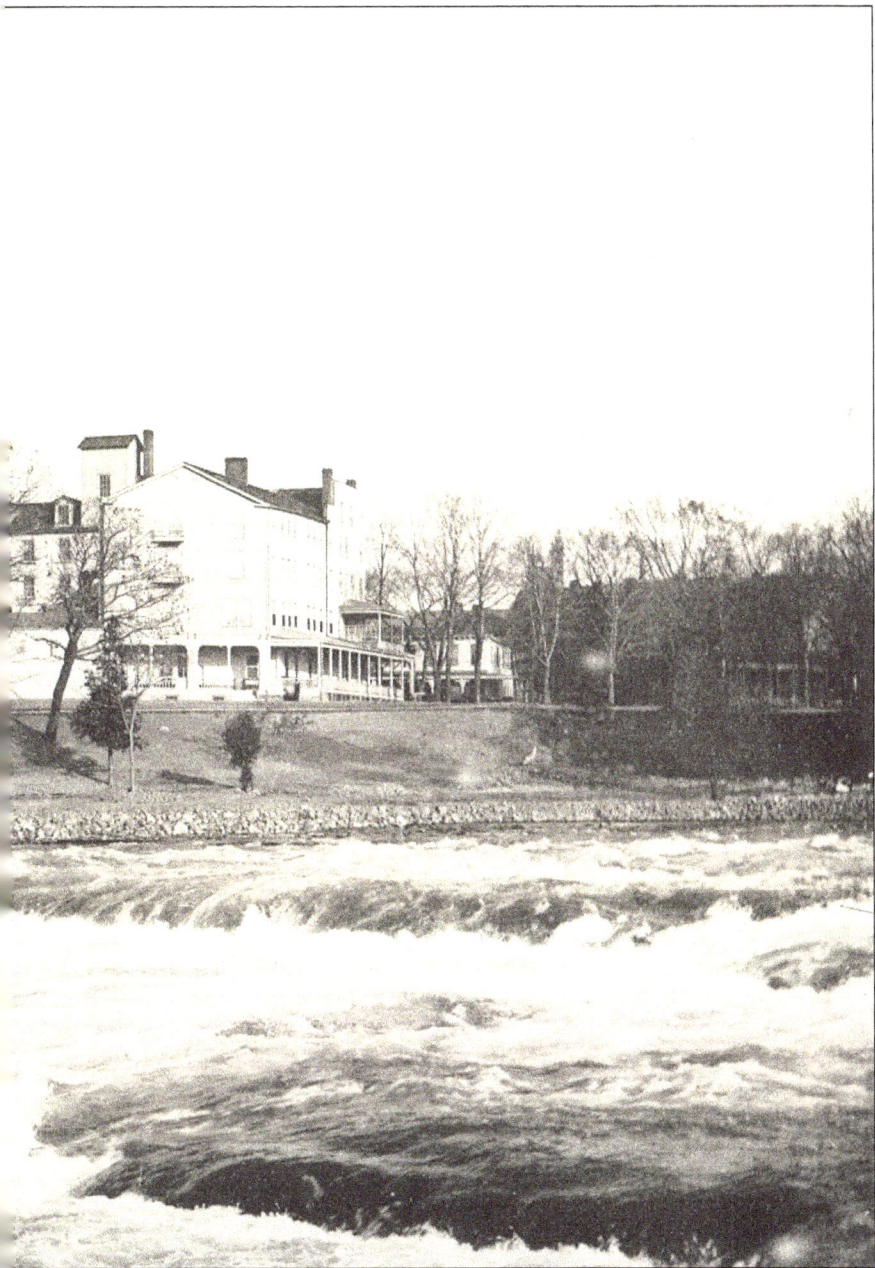

A November 12, 1900, article in *The Buffalo Express* once again brought attention to the former baths. A proposition was made to the Niagara Reservation Commission to revive the once popular current baths that operated above the Falls, but it was not implemented.

OLD CUSTOM MAY BE REVIVED

BATHHOUSE PLANNED FOR THE NIAGARA RAPIDS

CURRENT BATHING, ONCE POPULAR AT NIAGARA FALLS MAY BE RESUMED, IF THE RESERVATION COMMISSION GIVES ITS CONSENT.

Bathing in running water was years ago regarded as highly beneficial to cases of nervous disorders. Hundreds sought the Niagara baths from all over the country and it is probable that they were attracted there merely because of the name of the river. Such baths are held to be of value in nervous disorders, for imagination plays a large part in the cure of many such cases.

November 12, 1900, article in the *Buffalo Express*.

In 1945 the Cataract House Hotel, after serving as a training center and barracks for the Air Force during WWII, was destroyed by fire. Abraham Lincoln, General Ulysses S. Grant, Grover Cleveland, William McKinley, Millard Fillmore, Theodore Roosevelt, Edward VII of England, Mark Twain, and Charles Dickens were all famous guests of the hotel. You would wonder if they ever experienced the strong current baths.

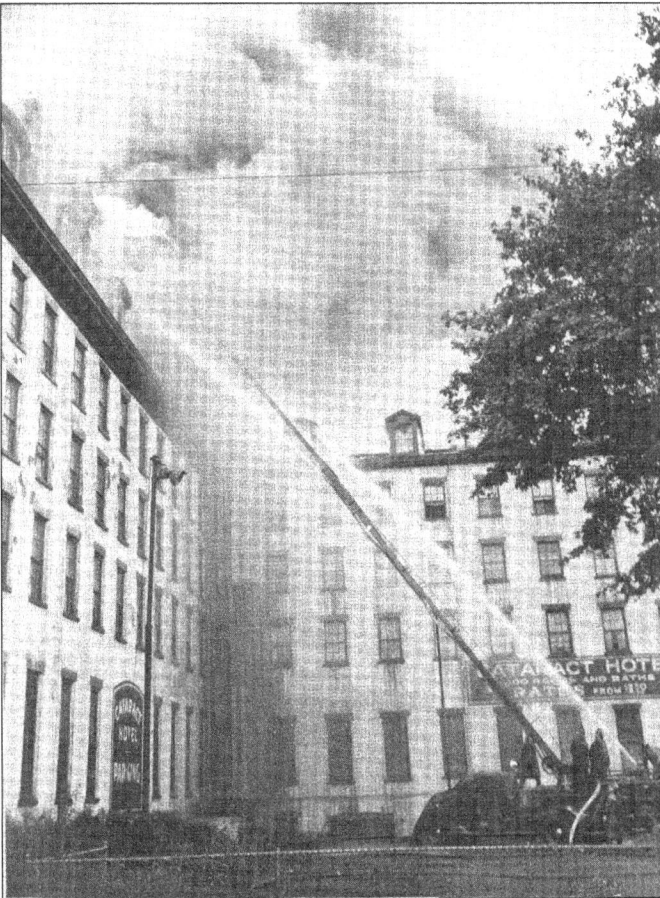

On October 14, 1945, the Cataract House was on fire and was unable to be saved. *Niagara Falls Gazette,* October 15, 1945.

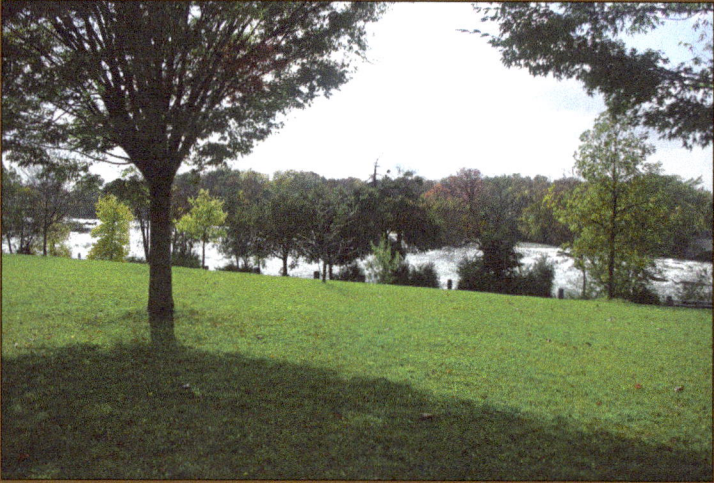

What's there now?

Former location of the Cataract House. View from the Robert Moses State Parkway. Niagara Falls, NY.

The River Hotel
(River Parlor Bath House)

This hotel was built by Mr. Tugby, and the building was expanded several times. The upper stories were a hotel, and the lower area contained a bathing house. Like the Cataract House, the River Hotel used the force of the rapids to provide a strong current bath to the guests. Among the operators of the hotel were J.V. Carr, J.T. Fulton, Mr. Behr, Frederick Jacobs, R.W. Jacobs, and Whitney and Jerauld & Co. The property had a variety of names: The International Hotel, the River Hotel, the Goat Island Hotel, the River Parlor Bath House and the Behr Hotel.[5] It was located just before the bridge to Bath Island (now Green Island). The Hotel offered warm showers and strong current baths.

The River Parlor Bath House was on an adjoining lot close to the Cataract House Hotel. The River Hotel was where the majority of the "strong current baths" were found. The two hotels were often marketed together and periodically managed as one unit. To the average tourist or travel writer, both may have appeared to be part of the large Cataract House Hotel complex.

As a result of the Niagara Commission efforts to restore the area around Niagara Falls, the River Hotel was sold in 1885 and the materials were used to build a restaurant on the Canadian side of Niagara Falls.

When the River Hotel property was catalogued for purposes of the Niagara Reservation Commission in 1885, it was listed as "The Cataract Hotel Property, known as the River Parlors and Ball-Room-Sold."[6]

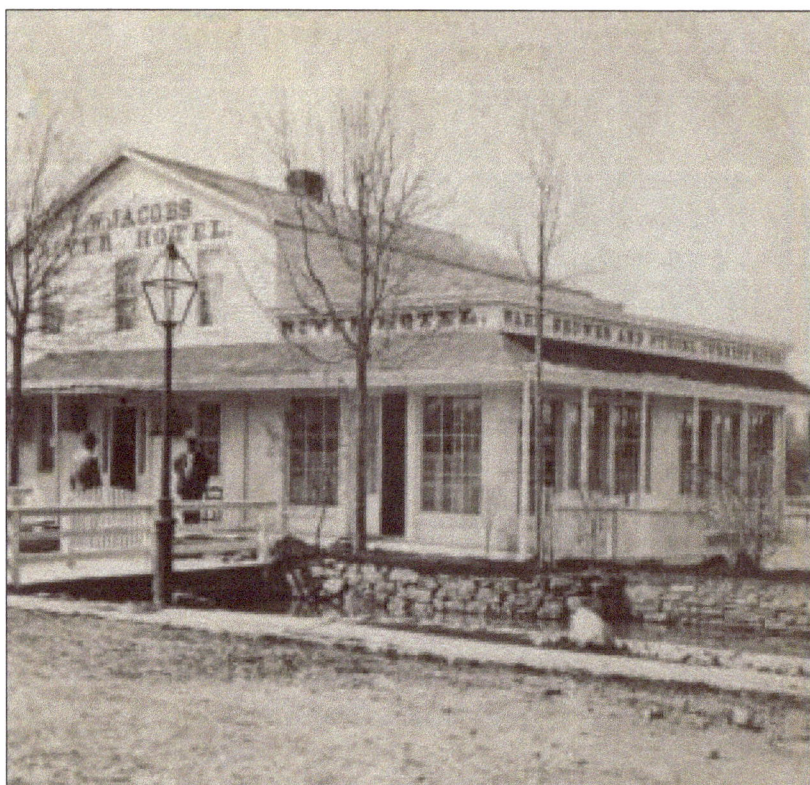

Image of the River Hotel, operated by R. W. Jacobs, which highlights the strong current baths.

CHAPTER 4

Health Products of Niagara Falls, NY

The Petrified Spray of the Falls

This was a substance that seemed unique to Niagara Falls and there are claims that it was used by Native Americans for medical purposes to cure open sores, skin problems, and malignant ulcers. Niagara Falls is documented as an early trade center for Native Americans and early explorers, and the petrified spray was one of the main objects of trade among the Native American tribes.[1]

Also called "Erie Stones," they were initially collected at the base of the falls and according to Robert McCauslin, MD, who wrote a 1789 scientific paper titled "An Account of an Early Substance Found Near the Falls of Niagara and Vulgarly Called the Spray of the Falls," the petrified spray stones were not found above the Falls—the majority were located at the base of the Falls and none were found at one mile or more from the Falls.

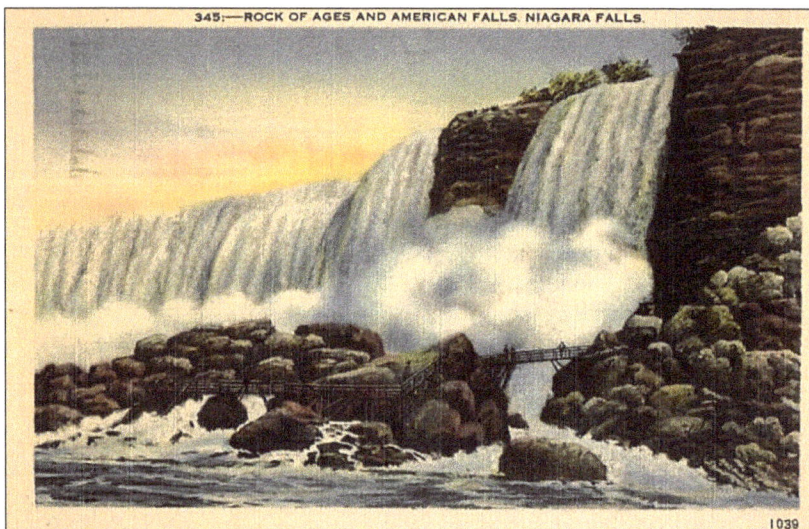

Petrified spray of the Falls. An early researcher believed that the majority was to be found below the falls.

This was part of Dr. McCauslin's ongoing studies into the historic recession of the Falls. Dr. McCauslin lived in Niagara Falls very close to his interests.

According to a 1985 paper presented to the Ontario Archaeological Society London Chapter, the "petrified spray" or "Erie Stones" were the mineral aragonite. This "stone" is found on the walls of the Niagara Gorge as a result of water seeping through beds of limestone. The paper then states:

> "Below the dolostone layer is a shale layer known as the Rochester shales. The water seepage does not penetrate through this layer, so it flows horizontally along the layers of dolostone which outlet at the Niagara gorge and run down the side of the rock face. Because of the evaporation of some of the water, calcium carbonate and the mineral aragonite are produced (Murphy 1982:

personal communication). Contrary to the theory of many of the visitors to the gorge, it is not the spray from the falls that has created this mineral. In some localities along the gorge the buildup of aragonite amounts only to a small film on the wall, but in other localities it builds up to four or five centimeters and appears as a frothy greyish looking stone."

The buildup on the gorge walls could be up to 1.5 to 2 inches. The scientific paper continues with a chapter titled "Curative Value":

> "The current therapeutic use of aragonite as outlined in contemporary medical journals indicates that calcium and magnesium were extremely useful in treating osteoporosis, leg cramps in pregnancy, improvement in breast milk, preventing premature birth, and the treatment of ulcers. An increase in calcium and magnesium in the diet may have been recognized by the Indians as a means of improving health and perhaps even the health of pregnant women."[2]

For the tourist industry, Native Americans and other vendors began to fashion jewelry and beads out of the petrified spray and other forms of gypsum that were available and better suited as raw material for their products.

As the tourist business increased, the stones were eventually imported from outside the area, with the majority imported from Wales, Great Britain, and sold by Native Americans and souvenir shops in the form of jewelry or powder in a small sack hung around the neck. A Dare Devil Barrel necklace was a favorite. The product claimed good health and good luck for wearers.

In the early 1900s the Dare Devil Barrel became a symbol of the dare devils of Niagara Falls. It was believed that the barrel would bring the good luck that schoolteacher Annie Edson Taylor had when she survived a trip over the falls in a barrel in 1901.

Even today there are health claims for selenite, a soft, glossy form of gypsum found in Niagara County. It's believed that contact with selenite will give you mental clarity, access to angelic guidance, energy, and assistance with balancing your relationship with the universe. The Internet has many shops offering selenite and dozens of claims for its benefits.

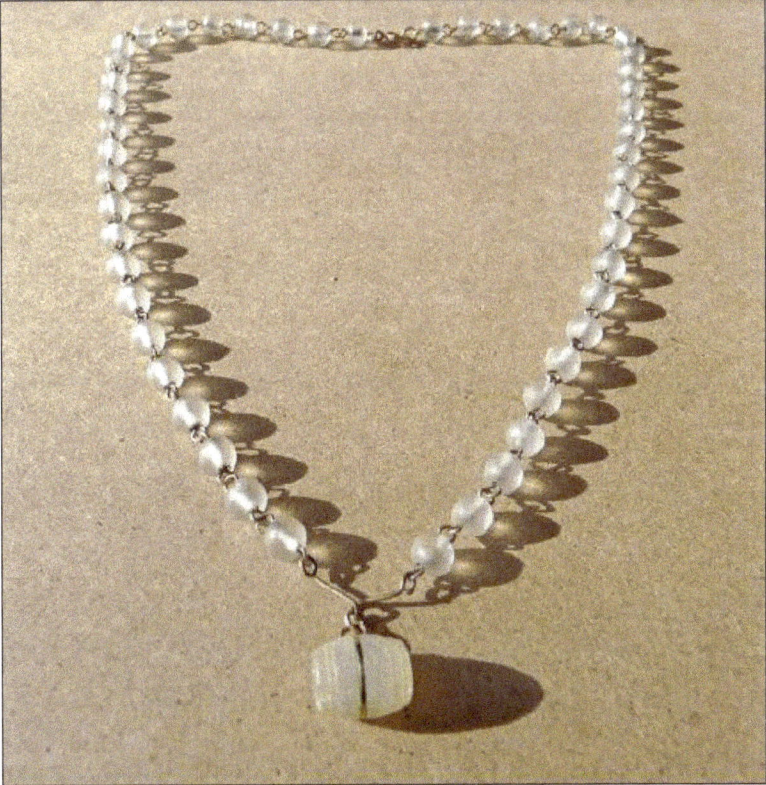

Antique petrified spray of the Falls with Dare Devil Barrel, and in the barrel, a Stanhope viewer of the Falls. Collection: J Boles

American Electro-Neurotone Company (1898–1901) Niagara Falls, NY

This electronic device manufacturer was located in the Niagara Falls Hydraulic Power and Manufacturing Complex that Jacob Schoellkopf owned. It was at the corner of Whirlpool and Chasm streets. The company produced an electronic apparatus that was used in Electro-Therapy medical treatments, the Hodgkinson's Electro-Neurotone. The machine claimed to cure rheumatism, nervousness, neuralgia, paralysis, sprains, dyspepsia, sciatica, stiff joints, constipation, lumbago, and spinal irritation. The business operated in 1898 under the leadership of F. W. Christie.

Although it opened in 1898 with considerable publicity, the Niagara Falls Business Directory does not list it after 1901. Newspaper articles from 1898 mention that the company operated in eight countries. The Electro-Neurotone Machine was patented by T. G. Hodgkinson. In the 1930s the company's main headquarters was in London, England.

ELECTRO NEUROTONE

United States Patents, 500-539
The new ELECTRO MASSAGE

The most unique, effective, simple, successful
in treatment of Neuralgia, Sciatica, Paralegia,
and the after effects of Paralysis. Endorsed
by highest authorities in the United States,
England and Canada. Manufactured only by
The American Electro-Neurotone Co.

Send for Treatise.
Niagara Falls, NY.

Advertisement placed in *Charlotte Medical Journal* (Volume v.13,
1898: July-Dec.)

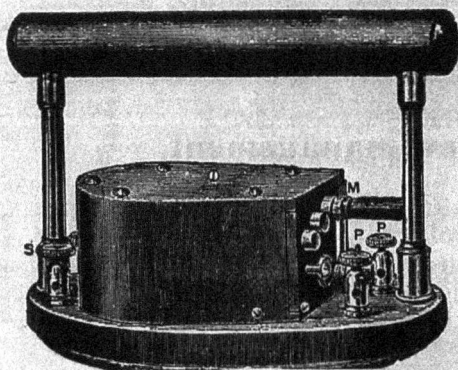

ELECTRO=NEUROTONE

United States Patents, 500--539.

The new
ELECTRO=MASSAGE
APPARATUS

The most unique,
" " effective,
" " simple,
" " successful
in treatment of Neuralgia, Sciatica, Paraplegia, and the after
effects of Paralysis.

Endorsed by highest authorities
in the United States, England
and Canada.

The American Electro-Neurotone Co.,
NIAGARA FALLS, N. Y.

The American Electro-Neurotone Electro-Massage Apparatus,
manufactured in Niagara Falls, NY.

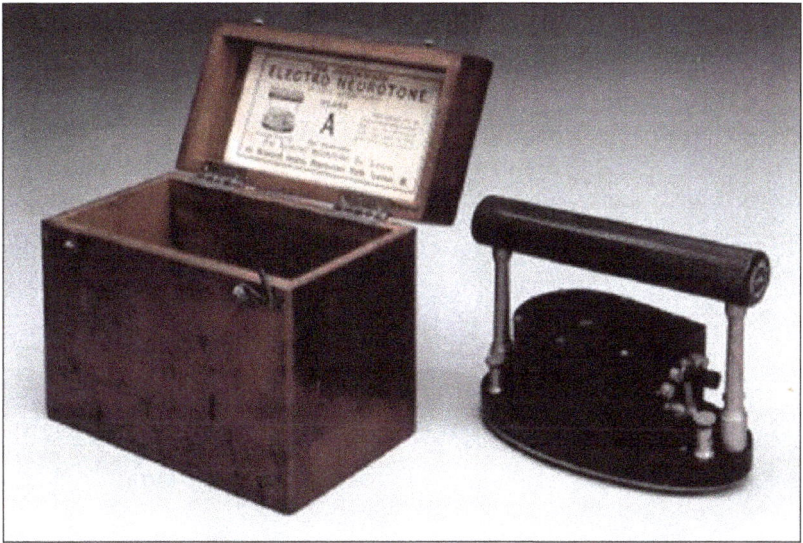

A newer version of the electro-neurotone appliance. This was manufactured in London, England, in the 1920s.[3]

THE HODGKINSON ELECTRO NEUROTONE.

Is the most efficient Electro Massage appliance in the treatment and cure of Neuralgia, Sciatica, Rheumatism, Nervous Prostration, Stomach Diseases, Insomnia, various forms of Paralysis, Neurasthenia or Spinal Irritation, etc.

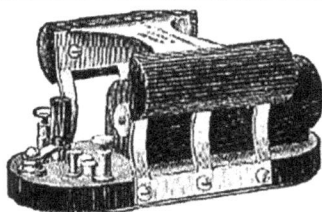

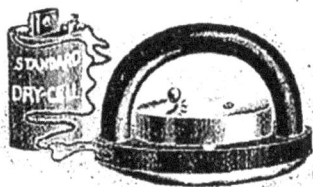

Class O, Physician's, with Cords and Dry Battery, in Case, $12.00.

The Electro Neurotone is cleanly, portable, reliable. No wet sponges, no sloppy batteries, no shocks. It is a recognized curative agent, destined by merit and good opinion to supersede many of the so-called electrical "cure-alls" of the present day.

Physicians who wish to prescribe a Medical Battery for a patient will find the Electro Neurotone fills every requirement.

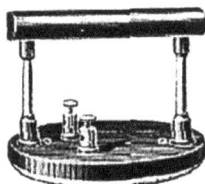

Class X, Neurotone in Case, with Dry Cell and Cords, $6.00.

The successful results which have attended the use of Neurotone apparatus when applied in cases of severe Sciatica, or in Paraplegia or Rheumatoid Arthrites and the varied after effects of Paralysis are largely due to the combination of the "D" instrument with the Neurotone. The facility with which nerves can be stimulated throughout their course— or muscular troubles overcome—presents numberless opportunities for demonstration.

The sole right to manufacture Electro Neurotone Apparatus in the United States is controlled by

Class D, Extension Instrument for Fixed or Movable Treatment, $6.25.

THE AMERICAN ELECTRO NEUROTONE CO.,
Niagara Falls, N. Y.

ALL ARTICLES DESIGNATED BY A * ARE ILLUSTRATED.

This device passed a weak electric current over the affected area.
The Hodgkinson Electro Neurotone manufactured in Niagara Falls, NY.
Niagara Falls Gazette, 1897.

What's there now?

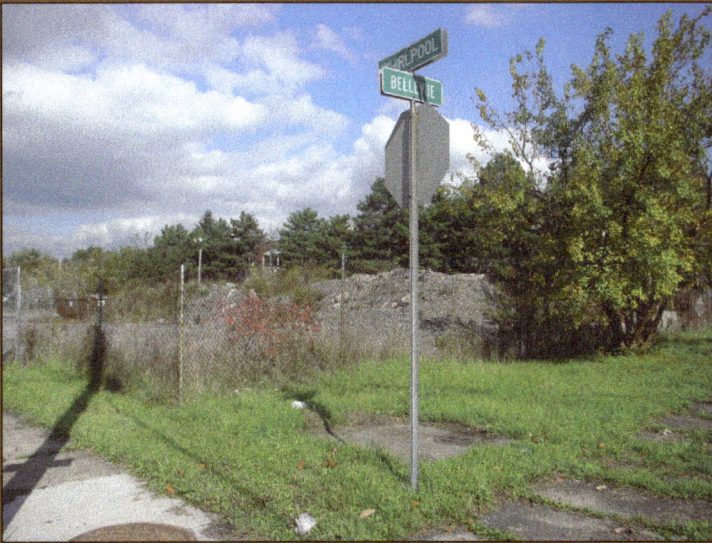

Corner of Whirlpool Street and Chasm Street. Former location of the American Electro-Neurotone Co., 1899, Niagara Falls, NY.

The Natural Food Conservatory (The Shredded Wheat Company)

In 1901, because of the inexpensive available electric power and the powerful image of Niagara Falls as a force of nature, the Natural Food Conservatory moved its operations to Niagara Falls, NY. The factory was known as the Palace of Light with white tile, bright lights, and many amenities for workers. It was built overlooking the rapids of the Niagara River.

The company was a progressive employer with a free hot lunch, rest breaks, air conditioners, showers, and a health and welfare fund that covered sickness, injury, and burial expenses.

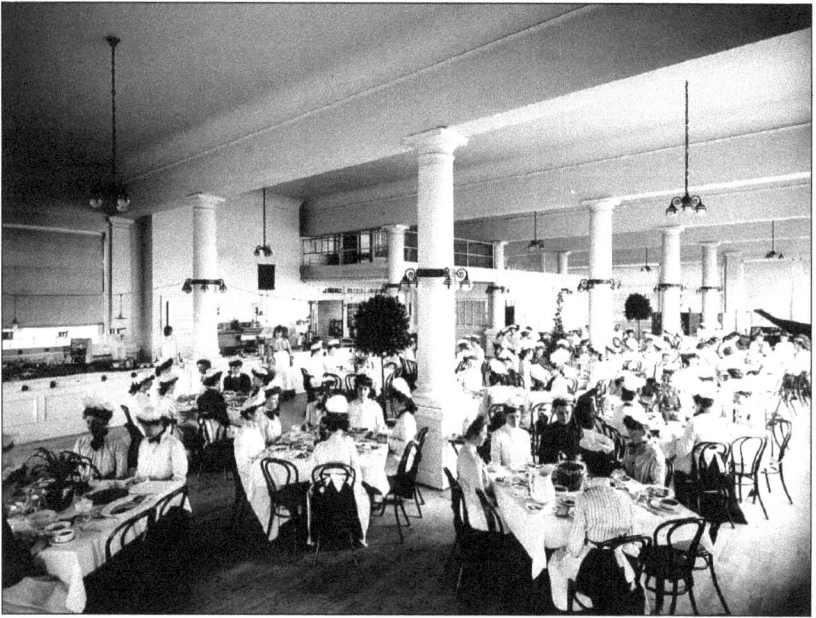

Ladies Lunch Room at the Natural Food Conservatory.

The name was changed to the Shredded Wheat Company in 1908. Although the company had many factories, the Niagara Falls building was very well known because of its promotion as a tourist attraction, with thousands of visitors per year.

The early history of the company goes back to 1895 in Worcester, Massachusetts. Known as the Cereal Machine Company, the products sold were Granulated Wheat-Shred, Wheat-Shred Drink, Shredded Cereal Coffee, Wheat-Shred Baby Food, and Shredding Machines.

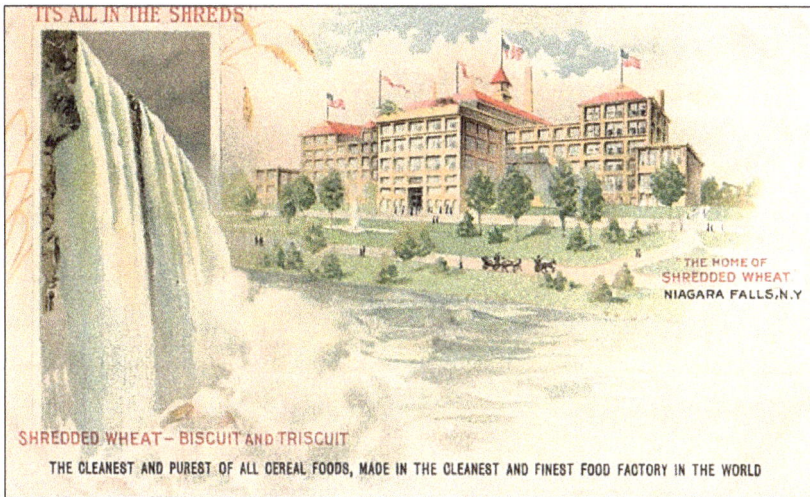

The "Palace of Light" with the natural image of Niagara Falls.

In Niagara Falls the main products were Shredded Whole Wheat Biscuit and Triscuit.

The list of health benefits for Shredded Wheat and Triscuits included:

- Relief from constipation
- Promotes an active brain
- Use as a "spring tonic"
- Builds muscles and bone
- Repairs waste tissues
- Builds strength
- Clear complexion
- Healthy teeth
- An entirely healthy body
- Brain making

Ad in *Good Housekeeping*, April 1929.

A 1903 Ad from *Current Literature*, August.

Mabel Lucie Attwell series promotional leaflet from the early 1920s. Attwell was a British illustrator famous for magazine illustrations.

Early Ad from the Natural Food Company. Niagara Falls, NY.

In 1963 parts of the "Palace of Light" on Buffalo Avenue were demolished. For a time, the remaining office building was used by Niagara County Community College as a college office and classrooms. The building was demolished in 1976.

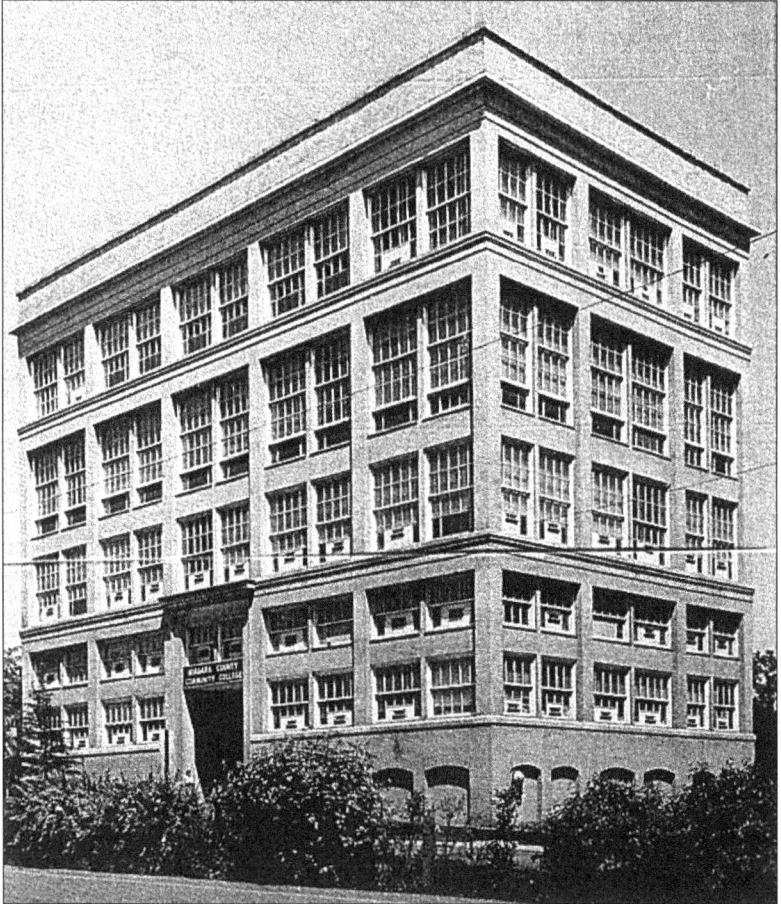

Old Shredded Wheat building at 430 Buffalo Avenue, Niagara Falls, NY. Also known as "Nabisco U" because it was used by Niagara County Community College in the 1960s and 1970s.

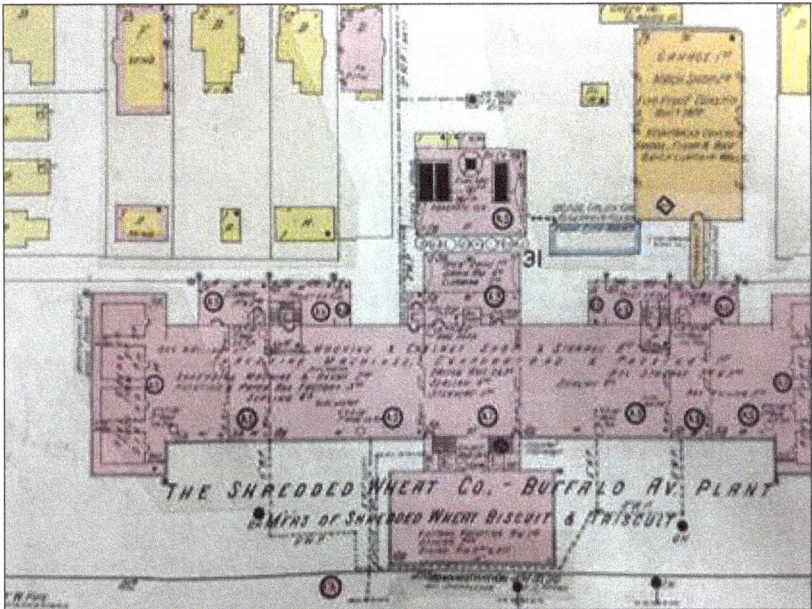

The Shredded Wheat Company. 1914 Sanborn Fire Map.

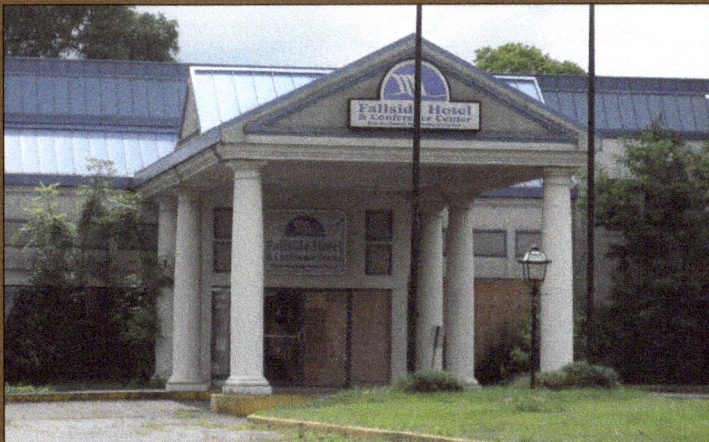

What's there now?

This is the former location of the Shredded Wheat Company. Fallside Hotel and Conference Center, 401 Buffalo Avenue, Niagara Falls, New York. Now closed.

Yeast-Vite Compound (USA) Inc., Beecham's Pills, and Beechalax

These three British medicines were marketed together and distributed by the Thomas Beecham Company, Lancashire, England.

Yeast-Vite Compound

A medicine marketed for the relief of headache and nerve pains, the company's United States address was Canal Basin, Niagara Falls, NY, and 904 Buffalo Avenue in Niagara Falls.

S-1129. *Yeast-Vite.* J. A. Johnson, New Haven. Yeast Vite (U.S.A.), Inc., Niagara Falls, N.Y. Declared. grains per tablet, acetphenetidin 0.37, found 0.42; amidopyrine declared 0.75, found 0.64; ammonium bromide declared 0.16, found 0.04; potassium bromide declared 0.21, found 0.34; caffeine declared 0.54, found 0.10; sodium bicarbonate declared 2.14, found 1.95; yeast declared 2.30, found present, amount not determined. Because of presence of amidopyrine can now be dispensed only on prescription, Sec. 17 (k).

Analysis of Yeast-Vite 1941. Now a prescription drug.[4]

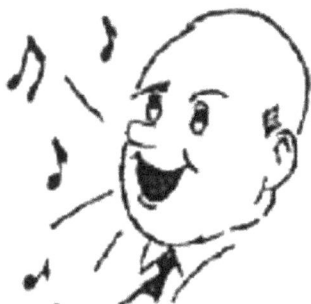

The Niagara Falls Gazette,
April 30, 1934.

Beecham's Pills, Niagara Falls New York, 1933–1935

Beecham's Pills were an English health product that, according to the Niagara Falls business directories, operated from 1933–1935 in Niagara Falls, NY. The address was listed as Hydraulic Canal Basin and 904 Buffalo Ave., Niagara Falls, New York.

The principals in the Niagara Falls operations were J. H. Howard, A. M. Robertson and R. G. Bloomfield. The pills were invented by Thomas Beecham about 1842 in St. Helens, Lancashire, England. They were produced until 1998.

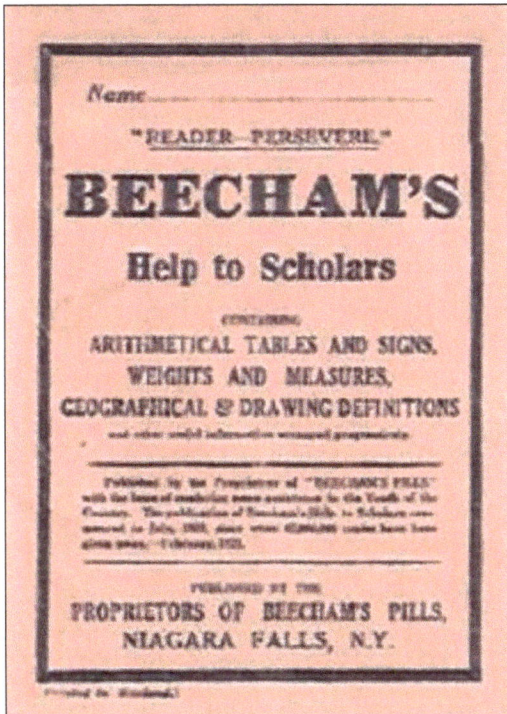

Beecham's Help to Scholars A Study Aid to students Geography, list of Presidents, math, states, and other school subjects. Beecham's Marketing, Niagara Falls, NY, 1929.

Beecham's Pills Ad in *Ladies Home Journal* listing both the New York City and English agents.

Beecham's claimed in its advertising that the pills would address the following problems:

- Female complaints
- Nervous disorders
- Constipation
- Consumption
- Disordered liver
- Depression
- Impaired digestion
- Bilious disorders
- Sluggish liver

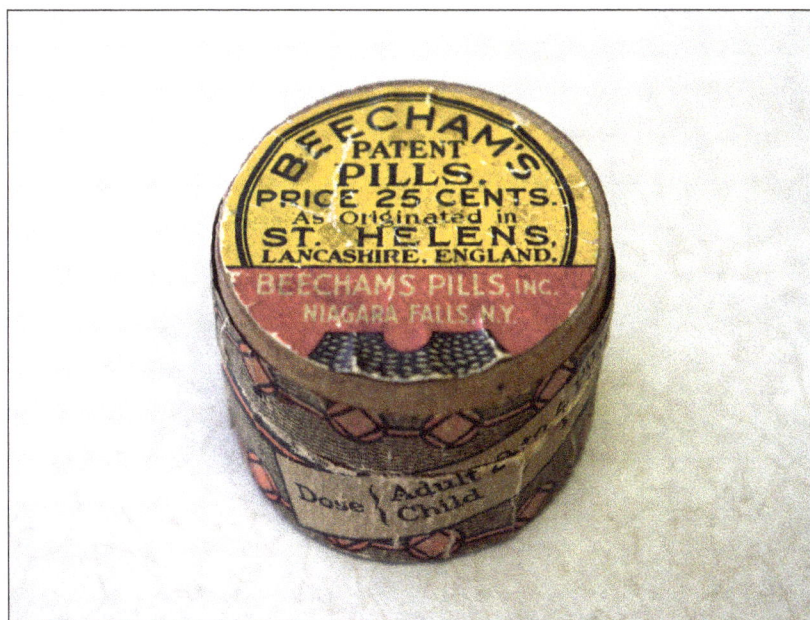

Beecham's Pills for bilious and nervous disorders. Manufactured in Niagara Falls, New York.

Beechalax

Beechalax was a strawberry-flavored laxative distributed by the Thomas Beecham Company, Lancashire, England. The company ads in 1934 stated the pills were manufactured in Niagara Falls, NY, at 904 Buffalo Ave.

All three of the British products were manufactured in Niagara Falls, NY. Ad from *The Niagara Falls Gazette*, January 2, 1934.

CHAPTER 5

Other Springs

Our research located a number of springs in the Niagara Falls area, and we believe there are many more along the Niagara Gorge and escarpment. Some of these springs and waters were mineral; others may have been clear water springs. These springs are listed to assist in any future research. For many there was very little information other than a brief mention in a newspaper or book.

Initial research on the waters of Niagara Falls centered on just the mineral springs or those with medicinal claims. However, it was decided to include all springs because readings indicated springs were generally regarded as being healthful and always a better alternative to city water or city wells. Also, there were health claims for springs that may have not been mineral springs. Even when officials determined a spring to be contaminated, they were still visited by residents. A good example of this is the well-known Goat Island Spring, which was declared unfit for drinking water several times and yet continued to be used. When it was stated by a local authority that Goat Island Spring was just river water, it remained a popular spring. Bottled, clear, or mineral spring water was an item in demand and there were many local bottlers to supply that need.

Goat Island Spring (Iris Island)

One of the best known of the public springs was the Goat
Island Spring located on the Niagara River on Goat Island,
which is on the brink of the falls. This spring was used
annually by thousands of tourists, the local hotels and
restaurants. Columbia Oak European Hotel, Rapids House,
Watson House, Mitchell's Restaurant, and Neidharts
Restaurant are mentioned in a 1910 study of local springs
as using the Goat Island water. The city of Niagara Falls had
frequent problems with its city water as it became "roily" or
muddy, so residents and businesses would use the Goat Island
Spring for clear water.[1]

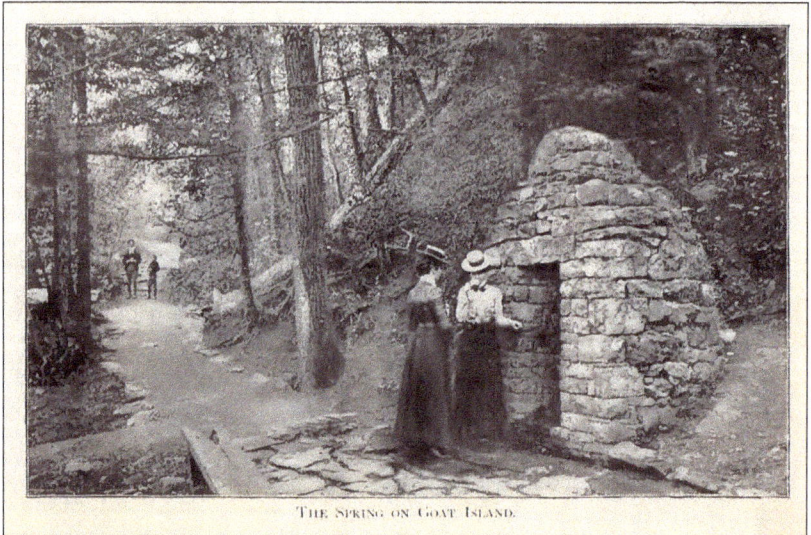

THE SPRING ON GOAT ISLAND.

Goat Island Spring, Niagara Falls, NY 1901.

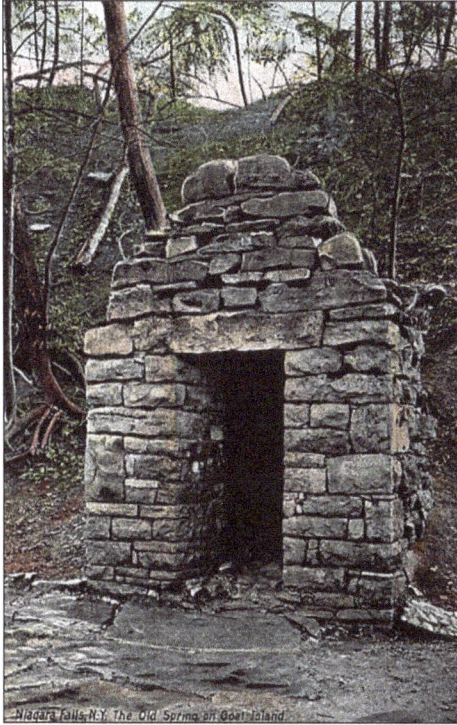

Early postcard view of the spring, titled
Niagara Falls, NY, Old Spring on Goat Island.

Around 1898, the city of Niagara Falls was experiencing an
outbreak of typhoid fever. A state expert was brought in that
year to investigate local wells and found "only two wells of 43
checked contained water fit for use. He also said the spring on
Goat Island was contaminated."

"The frame platform at the spring on Goat Island has been
removed, and the space floored with ledges of natural rock,
laid in sand. The Board of Health of the city of Niagara Falls
has called attention to the probable pollution of the water
by persons dipping pails and other vessels into the spring to
obtain water. To guard against possible contamination, it may
be well to close the opening in the stone canopy of the Spring,

so that the water may be obtained only through a tube."

A 1910 State Commissioner of Health report stated that "The spring is located in limestone which is greatly cracked and fissured. In all probability the water in the spring is river water that has entered by some fissure. The spring has never been known to run dry in summer. This water is used by a great number of people and, considering its geological features, its bacterial purity is questionable."[2]

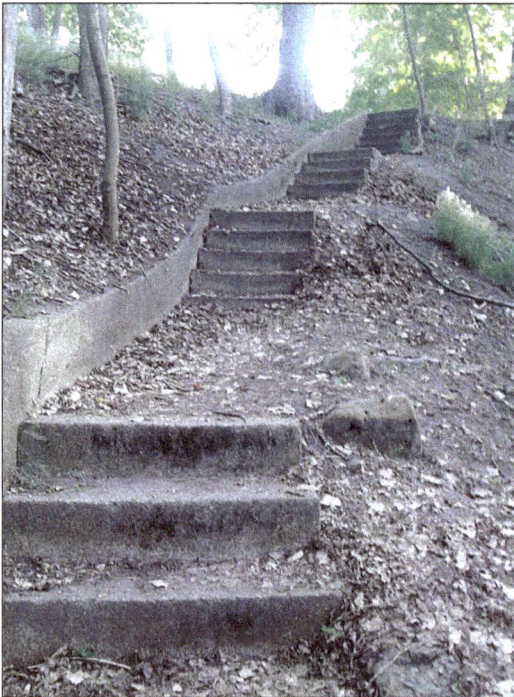

This spring is worth visiting. It is in a quiet area away from the falls and very close to the rapids. Today, stone steps lead to the Spring site. The Spring is located on the east side of Goat Island between the two bridges.
J Boles

Tonawanda - THE EVENING NEWS -
North Tonawanda

Thursday, October 1, 1914

The famous spring on Goat Island is to be
closed to the public. The water is reported to
be impure. There has long been a suspicion
that it is not a spring at all, but the outlet of
a stream of rock through which water from
Niagara River exudes.

1914 – Goat Island Spring closed to the public. The water was reported as impure. Also it was claimed that it was not a spring but water from the Niagara rapids running through a crack in the bedrock.

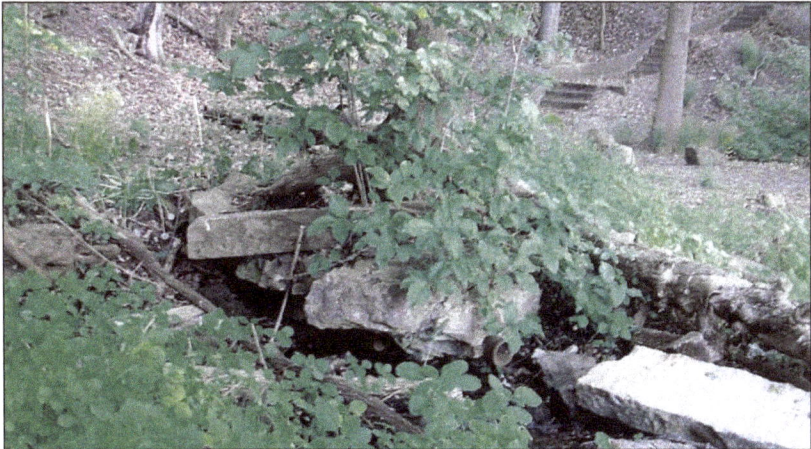

Remains of the Goat Island Spring with the stairs in the background.
J Boles

A present-day examination of the spring and the surrounding geology by a local geologist suggests that the spring is a true spring and not just river water forced through a fissure in the rock.

The Devil's Hole Cave Mineral Spring

This was a well-known and often visited spring because of the Great Gorge Route, a tourist railroad that ran along the gorge over the bridge to Canada, up the Canadian side of the gorge, and back across to the United States. The train would stop for passengers to explore the gorge or for a drink at the mineral spring, which was located in Devil's Hole Cave.

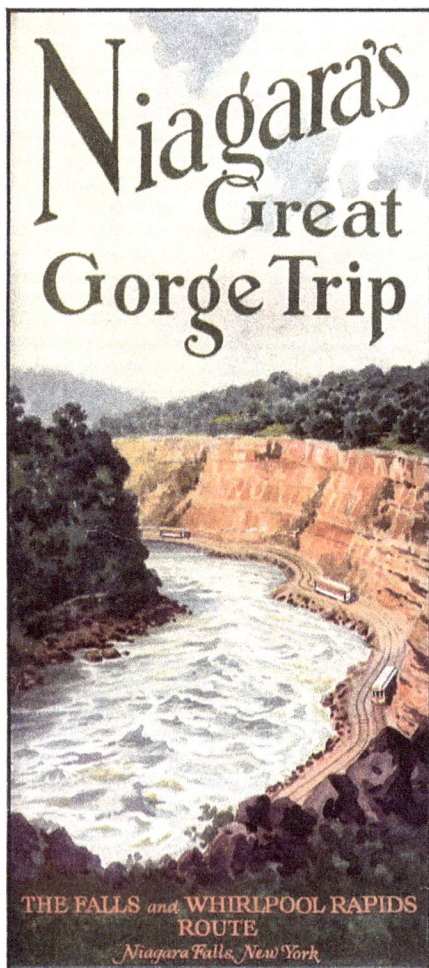

Niagara Gorge Railroad brochure.

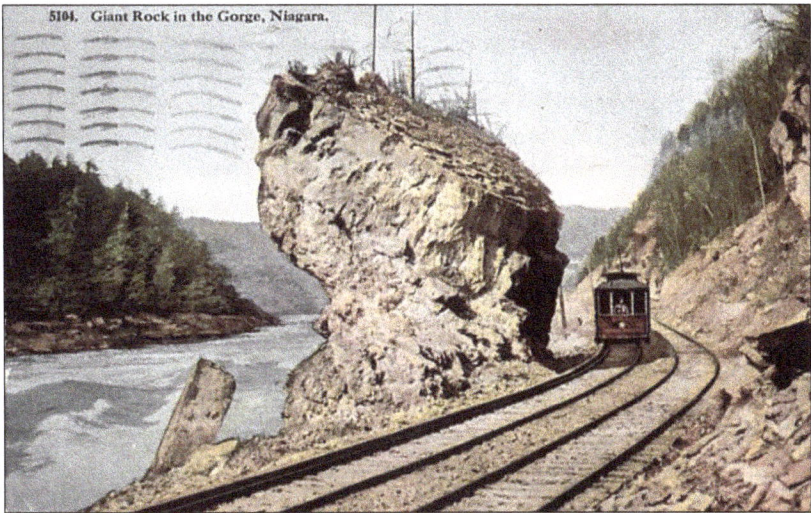

Niagara Gorge Railroad would stop at the Devil's Hole cave and mineral spring.

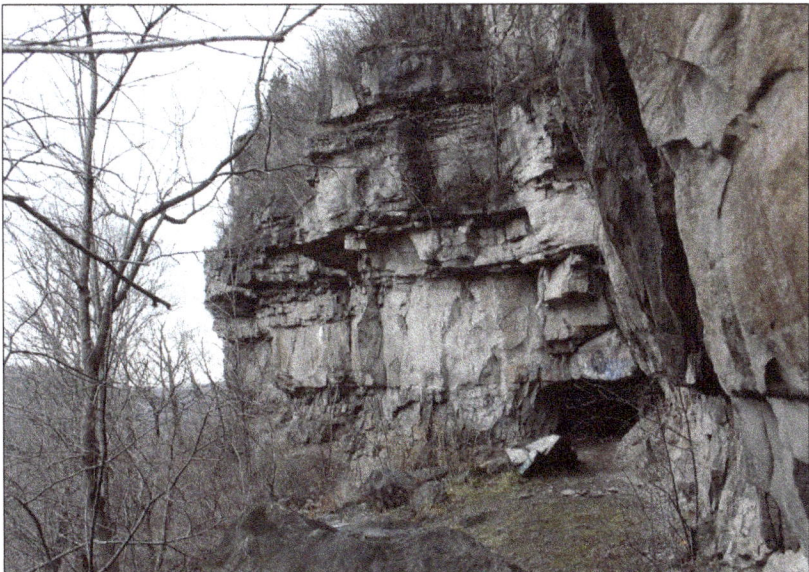

Devil's Hole cave entrance. The mineral spring flowed inside the cave.

It was originally nearly three-quarters of a mile in length. It contained three very large rooms which stood at right angles from the main hallway and were about 20 feet in width and 12 feet in height. Until 1854 this hole was in a perfect state of preservation. At that period a railroad made a deep cut diagonally over the main hallway. Their heavy blasting caused the rocks to fall and has closed the passage so that visitors should not attempt to go beyond the mineral spring. At the period when Europeans first visited this locality, the Devil's Hole was inhabited by the Neutral Nation of Indians and used by them as a hiding place in times of war. In order to keep their hiding place a secret, these Indians killed every person who entered the gorge at this point, and as these people never returned their friends came to regard this place as the home of the spirit of evil. In this way it naturally took its name, The Devil's Hole.

Description of Devil's Hole Cave and Mineral Spring. Niagara Gorge railroad pamphlet, "The story of the Devil's Hole."

This cavern is deeper than most others, and at the end of the spring of deliciously cool water issues from between two beds, the upper "spring line" of this region. There is no evidence that the cavern is extended any deeper than it does at present, nevertheless the spot is worth visiting, as it is the only accessible one of the numerous springs and caverns.

Guide to the Geology and Paleontology of Niagara Falls and Vicinity, 1901, by Amadeus William Grabau.

What's there now?

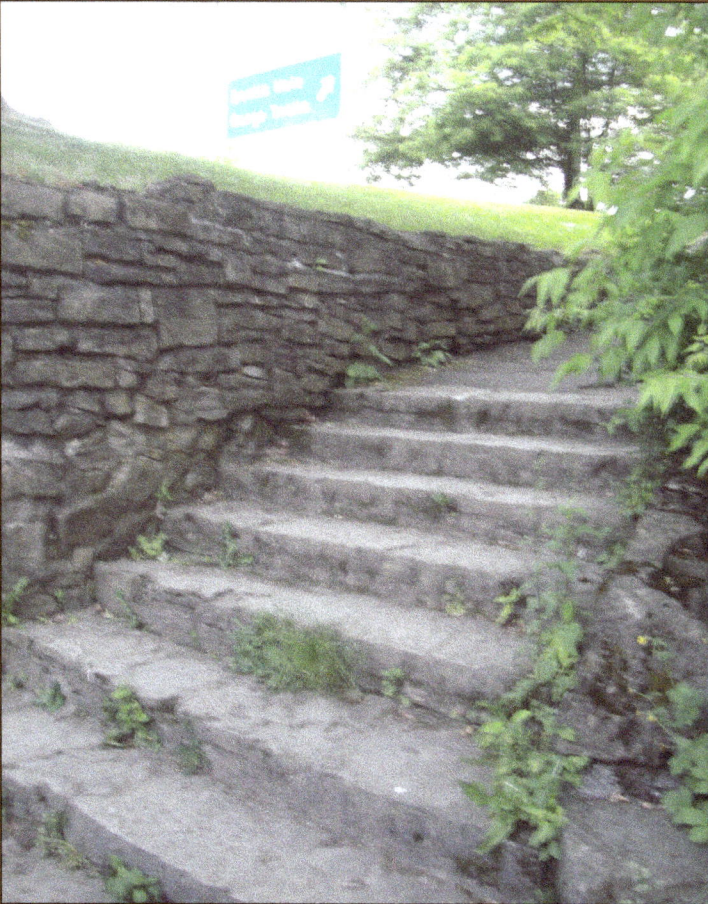

Stairs from the Devil's Hole parking lot leading to the Devil's Hole cave. Descending the stairs, the cave is to the right.

The Niagara Octagon Gas House and Spring (the Old Gas Station)

This unique structure built of red brick was located on Bellevue Avenue near the bank of the Niagara River. It was built in 1865 to provide gas to the North end and the Monteagle Hotel. A large steel tank collected gas while floating in a pool of spring water. Neighborhood children used to swim in the cold spring water. Later it was converted to a house and souvenir store.[3, 4]

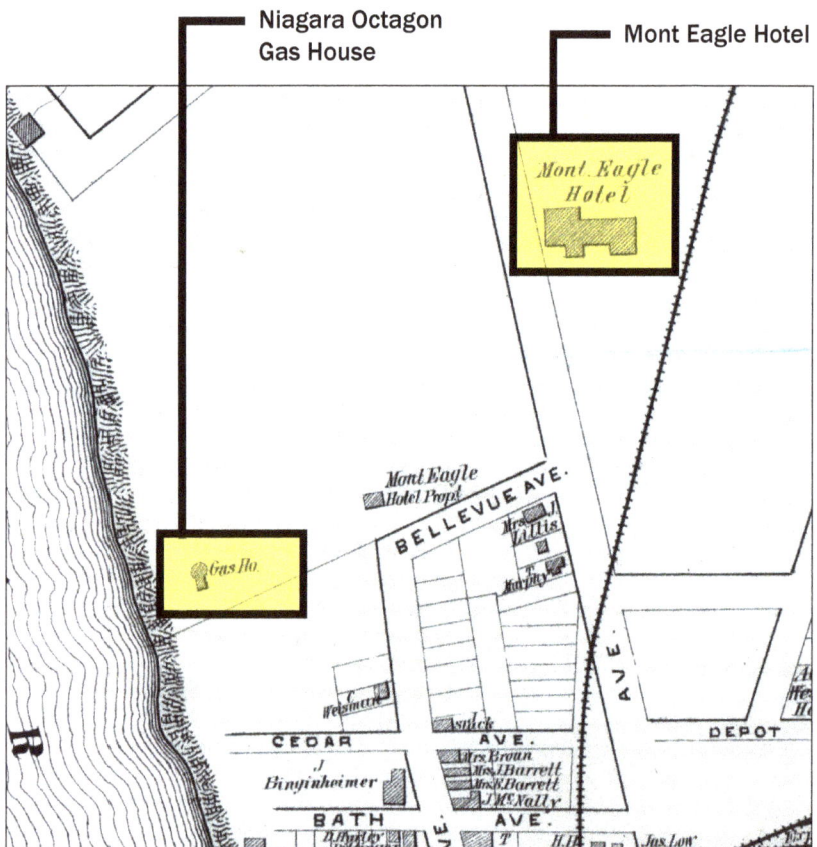

Niagara Falls, 1908, with the Niagara Octagon Gas House and the Monteagle Hotel indicated.

Lesser-Known Springs

1. Niagara Pharmacy Spring
- The Niagara Pharmacy was located at the Gluck Building at 203 Falls Street, Niagara Falls, NY. The Pharmacy sold natural mineral waters from American and European springs. There also was a spring in the basement of the pharmacy.

2. Cather's Cave and Mineral Spring
- Near Niagara Falls, NY
- Unimproved
- Calcic Lime Calcium Hydroxide - mineral water[5]

3. Catlin's Cave: Discovered by Mr. Catlin, Lockport, NY
- 194 feet southwest of the Schoellkopf Geological Museum, Niagara Falls, NY.

"The diameter of the cave is from 6-8 feet. It is of a circular form, having in its bottom a chrystal (sic) fountain of pure water. The entrance is a circular opening, that will admit the body of a medium size man."

Although listed in the United States Geological Survey as a mineral spring, there is no record of the water being bottled and sold. The cave and mineral spring were used as a tourist attraction with a fee charged to enter the cave. The cave and the spring were destroyed with the construction of the Schoellkopf hydro-electric plant.[6, 7]

4. Little Devil's Hole Spring
- In an early *Pocket Guide to Niagara Falls* (1842) the Little Devil's Hole Spring is mentioned.
- Location one quarter mile downstream from Devil's Hole.

- Little Devil's Hole Spring was "a strong mineral spring, impregnated with Sulphur." This spring was not located. It may have been destroyed by the construction of the power plant.

5. Niagara Falls Brewing Company
- Third Street near Cedar Avenue
- There were springs on the property

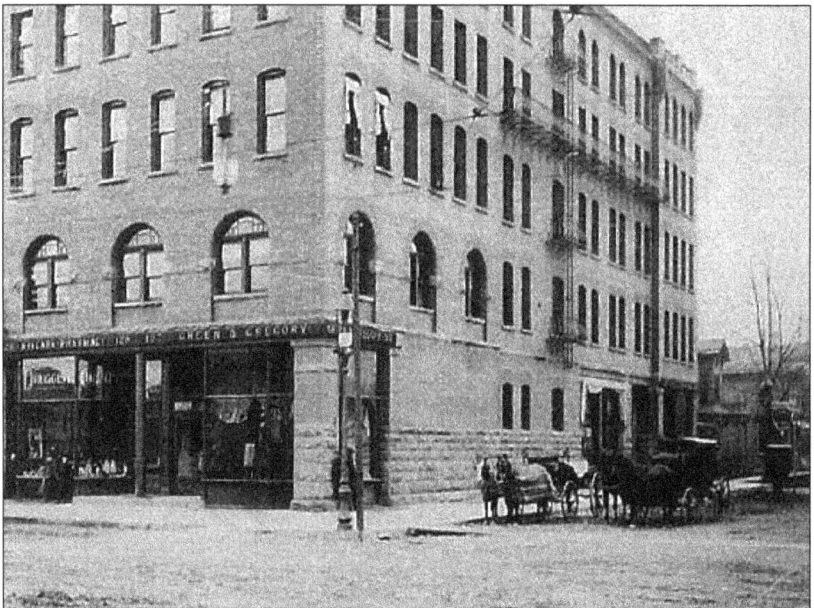

The Niagara Pharmacy: 2033 Falls Street, Niagara Falls, NY. The Pharmacy sold natural mineral waters from American and European springs. There also was a spring in the basement of the pharmacy.

CHAPTER 6

Bottling Works That Sold Mineral Waters

1. The Niagara Spring Water Company

LEHN ROCK SPRING WATER - An Excellent
drinking water, analyzed and highly recommended by
Herbert M. Hill, Ph. D., Chemist to city of Buffalo.
Sold by the Niagara Spring Water Co., 631 Pine Ave.
Bell Phone 1772.

This spring water was from the Lehn Rock Spring, Williamsville, NY.

2. Banks City Bottling Works

BANK'S CITY BOTTLING WORKS
CHARLES H. BANKS, MANAGER
Manufacturers and Dealers in all kinds of
Carbonated Beverages, Mineral Waters, Etc.
HOME PHONE 350. 552 SIXTH ST., NIAGARA FALLS, NY.

3. The Cold Spring Bottling Works

The Cold Spring Bottling Works,
458 Twenty-Sixth Street, Niagara Falls, N. Y.
Both Phones, Home, L183-Y, Bell 5133
Warehouse and Salesroom - 453 Nineteenth Street

4. Suspension Bridge Bottling Works

The Suspension Bridge Bottling Company operated from 1898 until 1955, according to business directories. The mineral water was last advertised as a product in 1911. The bottling plant was located at 712-716 Willow Avenue and later another plant was opened at nearby 829 Linwood Avenue.

The source of the mineral water is not known, however the bottling plant was close to the many mineral springs found in the Suspension Bridge area.

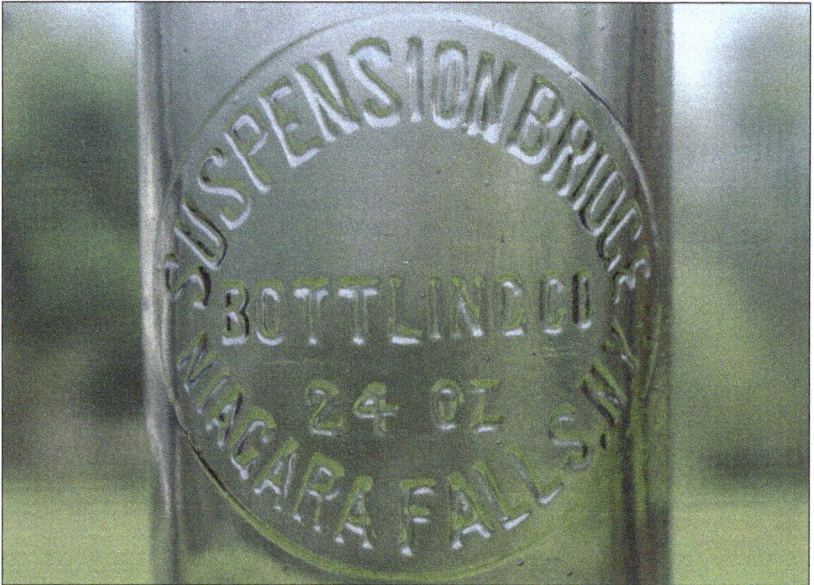

Suspension Bridge Bottling Company Bottle.

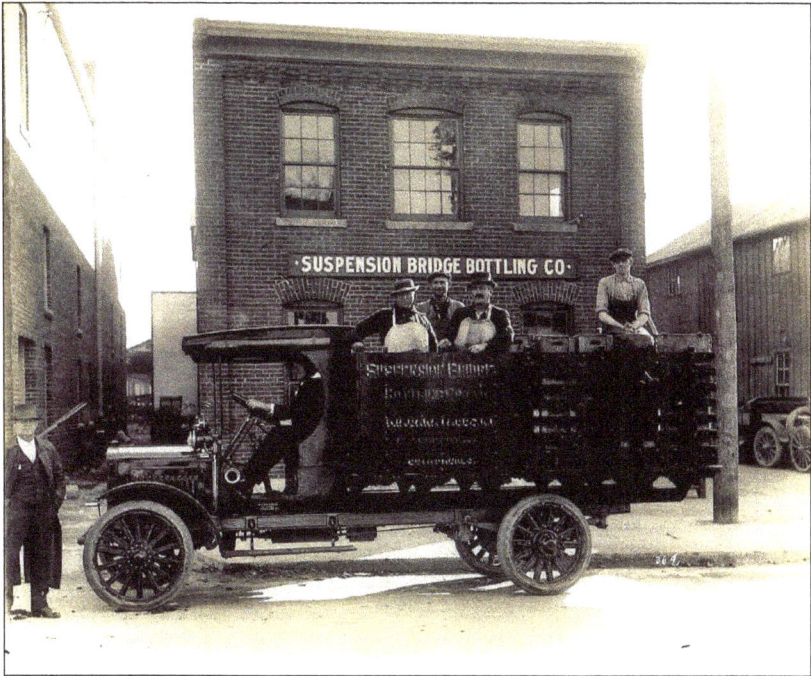

The Suspension Bridge Bottling Company, Former address 829 Linwood Avenue, present address 831 Linwood.

**SUSPENSION BRIDGE BOTTLING CO.,
BOTTLED FOR FAMILY USE**
Also Manufacturers of Ginger Ale, Soda
and Mineral Waters.

**SOLE AGENTS FOR
IROQUOIS BUFFALO LAGER**
712-716 Willow Ave.

What's there now?

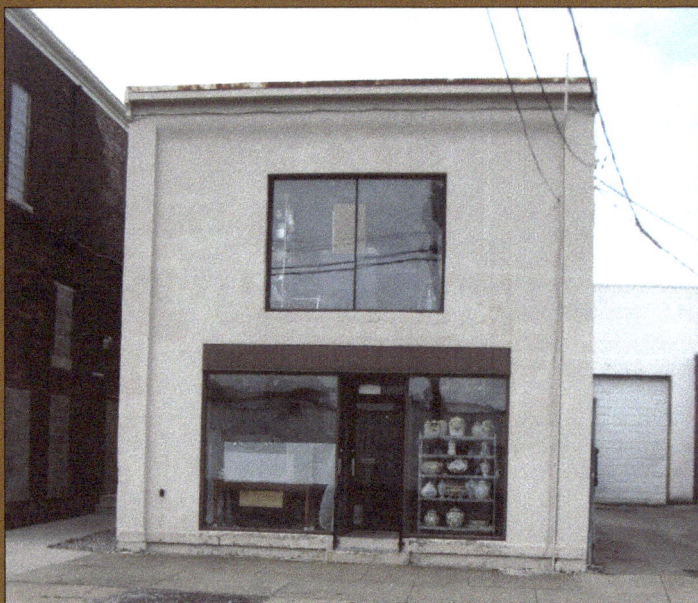

Former Suspension Bridge Bottling Company building. DiCamillo's Bakery Mail Order Business, 831 Linwood Avenue, Niagara Falls, New York. Thanks to David DiCamillo, DiCamillo Bakery, for the information on this building.

CHAPTER 7

Some Thoughts on Niagara Falls after Alternative Medicine Research

I t is possible that Niagara Falls would have been a
 successful mineral springs resort like Saratoga Springs, NY.
There were many springs located along the banks of
the Niagara River. However, the rapid-paced business
development with a focus on industrial power and the
construction of bridges, mill races above and below ground,

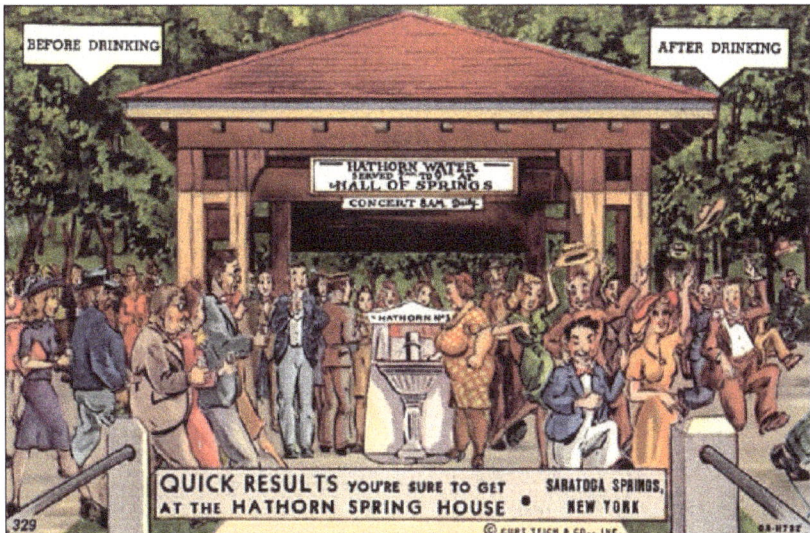

One of the many springs in Saratoga Springs NY. Note the quick results
after drinking the water.

> The mineral spring at Niagara Falls bids fair
> to become a place of much resort by the sick
> and invalids. It commands a fine view of the
> cataract, and its waters prove an officacious
> remedy in some diseases.

Geneva Gazette, Wednesday, June 13, 1829.

sewers, and buildings disrupted the spring activity. By the early 1900s, the springs that were concentrated near the Suspension Bridge were not viable and the spring-based hotels were used for other purposes.

The area was gifted with natural beauty, waterpower, then electric power, and ample water. Although the Niagara Commission restored some of the areas around the Falls, the city of Niagara Falls was constantly changed by manufacturing interests. It is a difficult area to research because many of the sites have been destroyed or altered.

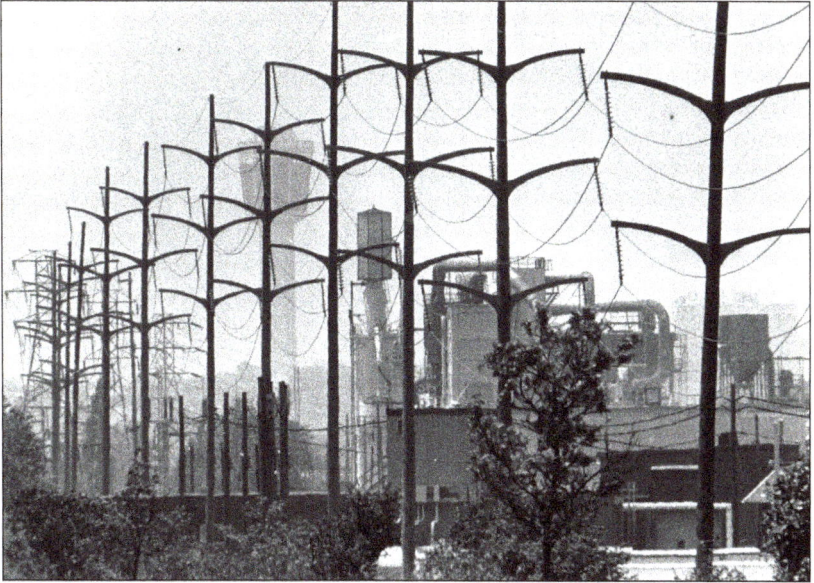

Niagara Falls, NY, industry and power.[1]

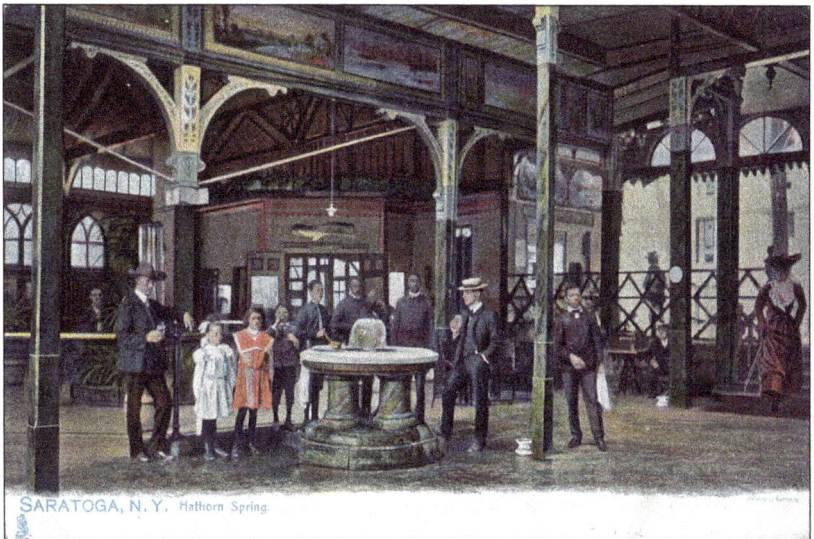

Hathorn Spring, Saratoga, NY. A successful spring-based resort town.

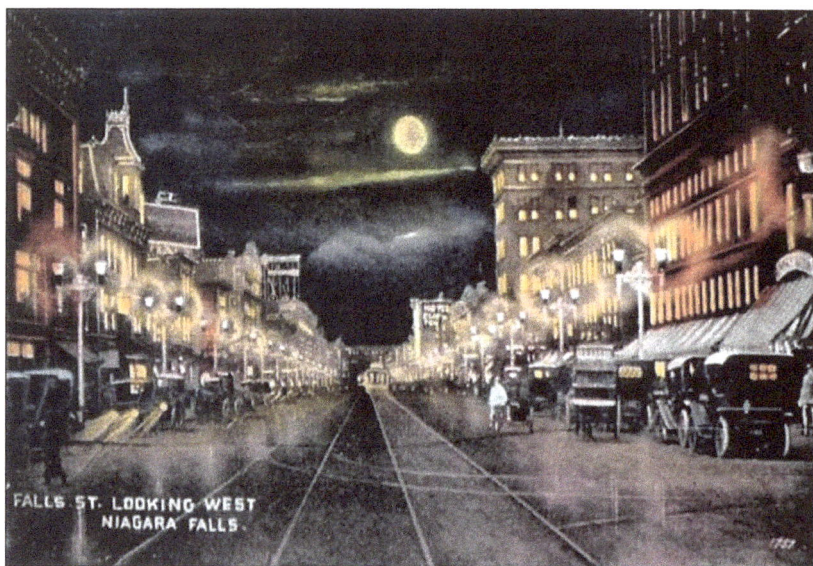

Early image of Niagara Falls as a tourist town.

Notes

Chapter 1:
1. *Suspension Bridge Journal* (May 10, 1884): 2.5.
2. *Niagara Falls Gazette* (March 1885)
3. *Suspension Bridge Journal* (December 31, 1887) 3.6.
4. http://en.wikipedia.org/wiki/Lithia_Springs,_Georgia (accessed 2014)

Chapter 2:
1. *Niagara Falls Gazette* (July 17, 1897).
2. *The Daily Palladium*, (December 28, 1897).
3. http://educate-yourself.org/fc/ (Accessed 2014)
4. *The Daily Cataract Journal* (May 13, 1901) 5.5.
5. *The Daily Cataract Journal* (May 22, 1901) 5.3.
6. *The Daily News* (May 5, 1902)
7. *Niagara Falls Gazette* (February 1926)

Chapter 3:
1. BGuthriePhotos. http://www.bguthriephotos.com/graphlib. nsf/keys/2007_NY_Niagara_FallsNY (accessed 2013)
2. http://images.library.pitt.edu/cgi-bin/i/image/image-id x?view=entry;subview=detail;cc=darlmaps;entryid=x-DARMAP0173;viewid=DARMAP0173.TIF (accessed 2013)

3. Gerry Biron. iroquoisbeadwork.blogspot.com (accessed 2013)

4. Niagara Falls, 1882, Birds Eye View, NY. H. Wellgedel. Beck & Pauli, 1882.

5. Judith Wellman. *Survey of Sites Related to the Underground Railroad, Abolitionism, and African American Life in Niagara in Niagara Falls and Surrounding Area 1820-1880.* 2012.

6. *The Buffalo Express* (November 1885)

Chapter 4:

1. Peter Porter. Niagara, *An Aboriginal Center of Trade.* Niagara Falls,1906.

2. James Hunter. *Newsletter of the London Chapter Ontario Archaeological Society.* Erie Stone: A 17th Century Iroquoian Medicinal Trading Commodity.

3. Image was found on Trademe.co.nz (accessed 2013), listing 574932871

4. The Forty-fifth report on food products and thirty-third report on drug products, *Connecticut Agricultural Experiment Station Bulletin* 447, Sept. 1941, pg. 447. Yeast-Vite was listed as produced in Niagara Falls, NY. In this report, the state of Connecticut has it classified as a prescription drug.

Chapter 5:

1. Thirty-First Annual NY State Dept. of Health, June 1910, pg 529.

2. Thirty-First Annual NY State Dept. of Health, June 1910, pg 530-531.

3. August 31, 1925, *The Niagara Falls Gazette.*

4. Daniel Davis (local Suspension Bridge Historian), in-person

interview by author, August 8, 2014.

5. Bulletin of the United States Geological Survey No. 32, Mineral Springs in NY, Washington Government Printing Office, 1886.

6. Scott Ensminger. *The Caves of Niagara County NY.* Number 27 of the Occasional Contributions of the Niagara County Historical Society, 1987.

7. Scott Ensminger, in-person interview by author, August 8, 2013.

Chapter 7:

1. *APN Sunday Illustrations*, 1883, New York, NY.

Acknowledgements

Thanks to all who helped with this publication.

Lois Crane

Susan Crocker

Rachel Bridges

Michelle Green

Danielle Herrmann

Sarah Jerge

Will Phillips

Rick Pope

Sallie Randolph

Melissa Royer

Stephanie Kryst Sullivan

Melissa Dunlap and
Anne Marie Linnabery
*Niagara County
Historical Society*

Daniel Davis
Niagara Falls, NY Historian

Katherine Emerson,
Craig Bacon and Ron Cary
*Niagara County
Historians Office*

Scott Ensminger

Larry Hasely, *Town of
Lockport Historians Office*

Lockport Public Library

Niagara Falls Public Library

Renee Printup, Neil Patterson
*Tuscarora Environment
Program*

Bibliography

Altman, Nathaniel, *Healing Springs: The Ultimate Guide to Taking the Waters.* Rochester, Vermont: Healing Arts Press, 2002.

Altman, Nathaniel, *The Spiritual Source of Life Sacred Water.* Mahwah, New Jersey: Hidden Spring Publishers, 2002.

Amato, Joseph A., *Rethinking Home. A Case for Writing Local History.* Berkeley and Los Angeles, CA: University of California Press, 2002.

Anderson, William J., *Hysterical and Nervous Affections of Women [A Paper].* Read before the Harveian Society. London: John Churchill, Princes Street, SOHO, 1853.

Armstrong, David and Elizabeth Metzger Armstrong, *The Great American Medicine Show, Being an Illustrated History of Hucksters, Healers, Health Evangelists and Heroes, from Plymouth Rock to the Present.* New York, NY: Prentice Hall, 1991.

Blumin, Stuart M. and Deborah Adelman Blumin. *The Short Season of Sharon Springs. Portrait of an American Village.* Ithaca, NY: Cornell University Press.

Bulletin of the United States Geological Survey. *Department of the Interior*, 32.

Carson, Gerald, *Cornflake Crusade*. New York, Toronto: Rinehart & Company, Inc., 1957.

Deutsch, Ronald M., *The New Nuts Among the Berries*. How Nutrition Nonsense Captured America. Palo Alto, CA: Bull Publishing Co., 1977.

Donegan, Jane B., *Hydropathic Highway to Health*. Women and Water-Cure in Antebellum America. Westport, CT: Greenwood Press, 1986.

Eichhorst, Hermann, *Handbook of Practical Medicine*. Woods Library of Standard Mecical Authors – Diseases of the Blood and Nutrition, and Infectious Diseases. New York, NY: Stettiner, Lambert & Co., 1886.

Gerstner, Patsy, *The Temple of Health*. A Pictorial History of The Battle Creek Sanitarium. Springfield, IL: Caduceus Volume 12, Number 2, 1996.

http://bguthriephotos.com

http://iroquoisbeadwork.blogspot.com by Gerry Biron.

Hunter, J. Newsletter of the London Chapter Ontario Archaeological Society. *Erie Stone: A 17th Century Iroquoian Medicinal Trading Commodity*.

Johnson, R. The Story of Medicine. *The Tuscarorans Mythology-Medicine-Culture, A Carolina Heritage Book*. Volume 1, 1967.

Lockie, L. *Pharmacy on the Niagara Frontier*. East Aurora, NY: Henry Stewart Incorporated.

McGreevy, Patrick, *Imagining Niagara*. The Meaning and Making of Niagara Falls. Amherst, MA: The University of Massachusetts Press, 1994.

Paris, Gloria, *A Child of Sanitariums. A Memoir of Tuberculosis Survival and Lifelong Disability*. Jefferson, NC: McFarland and Co. Inc., 1931.

Pierce, R. V. MD, *The People's Common Sense Medical Adviser*.

Buffalo, NY: The World's Dispensary Medical Association, 1918.

Porter, P. Niagara Falls 1906. In *Niagara, An Aboriginal Center of trade*. Retrieved from www.gutenberg.org

Prud'Homme, Alex, *The Ripple Effect. The Fate of Freshwater in the Twenty-First Century*. New York, NY: Scribner, 2011.

Niagara Falls Park a History. Retrieved from www. NiagaraFrontier.com

Ruck, Karl Von and Silvio Von Ruck, *A Clinical Study of Two Hundred and Ninety-Three Cases Treated at the Winyah Sanitarium, Asheville, N.C., in 1905 and 1906: With Special reference to Specific Medication and its Results*. LaVergne, TN, 2010.

Springer, A. & Stevens, L. Spheres of discharge of springs. *Hydrogeology Journal*.

Steiger, Brad, *Indian Medicine Power*. Gloucester, MA: Para Research, 1984.

The Broadway a London Magazine. Volume 1, September 1868-February 1869.

The Magazine of the Buffalo Museum of Science. (n.d.). *Minerals of the Niagara Frontier Region* [brochure]

Ensminger, Scott. The Caves of Niagara County New York. *The Niagara County Historical Society*, 27. 1987.

Definitions

Note: For historical accuracy, the exact language of the historical periods discussed in this book has been retained. No offense is intended toward any individual or group.

Aperture – a hole or opening through which light travels. (Wikipedia)

Catarrh – a disorder of inflammation of the mucous membranes in one of the airways or cavities of the body.

Cosmetic – skin care and conditions. (Wikipedia)

Cutaneous Afflictions – Skin infections. (Wikipedia)

Decline and General Prostration of Health – General decline in health and energy, run down. (Wikipedia)

Diagnostic – Serving to identify a particular disease. (Wikipedia)

Doctrine of Signatures – Nature had hidden clue to medically effective drugs. (Wikipedia)

Dyspepsia – a condition of impaired digestion. (Wikipedia)

Electro-Therapeutics – a general term for the use of electricity in therapeutics, i.e., in the alleviation and cure of disease. It is used as a treatment, like electroconvulsive therapy and TENS. (Wikipedia)

Erysipelas – a type of skin infection also known as St. Anthony's Fire. (Wikipedia)

Escarpment – a steep slope or long cliff that occurs from erosion or faulting and separates two relatively level areas of differing elevations. (Wikipedia)

Fissure – a groove, natural division, deep furrow, elongated cleft, or tear in various parts of the body. (Wikipedia)

Fistula – an abnormal connection or passageway between two epithelium-lined organs or vessels that normally do not connect. (Wikipedia)

Fragility – lacking physical or emotional strength. (The Free Dictionary)

Gout – a medical condition usually characterized by recurrent attacks of acute inflammatory arthritis—a red, tender, hot, swollen joint. (Wikipedia)

Homeopathic – treatment for diseases based on the administration of minute doses of a drug that in massive amounts produces symptoms in healthy individuals similar to those of the disease itself. (The Free Dictionary)

Hot Air Bath – exposure of the body to air and sun, without clothing; Victorian Tutors and more the Victorian Bathroom. (Wikipedia)

Hysteria – derived from the Greek word *hystera*, meaning "womb," and refers to a nervous disorder characterized by heightened emotional states, anxiety, and various mental alterations. Physicians long believed that hysteria resulted from a "disturbance in the womb," and thus confined the diagnosis exclusively to women. Because the symptoms could accompany a variety of other nervous disorders, hysteria was often applied to patients whose condition was otherwise unexplainable. Significant advancements in the understanding of hysteria occurred during the 1870s when a French neurologist named Jean-Martin Charcot conducted an in-depth study on three women admitted to the hysteria ward at the Salpêtrière Hospital in Paris. (*Gold Cures* book)

Invalid – a patient, a sick person; an archaic, politically incorrect term for a person with a disability. (Wikipedia)

Lumbago – a common disorder involving the muscles and bones of the back. (Wikipedia)

Mineral Bath – a bath that uses mineral water or minerals added. (Wikipedia)

Nerve Exhaustion – an American disease connected to our restless ambitions. If Nerve Exhaustion was not caught in its early stages, doctors felt that a general complete nerve breakdown would occur. Conditions included: fatigue, anxiety, headache, neuralgia and a depressed mood. Researchers at that time believed that furthering the tendency to this disease was the dry climate, extreme temperatures, civil and religious liberty, and the heightened mental activity of women. (*The Gold Cure Institutes of Niagara Falls, NY, 1890s*)

Neuralgia – pain in the distribution of a nerve or nerves. (Wikipedia)

Osteopath – a physician who was trained in the field of "osteopathic medicine." Osteopathic medicine emphasizes the whole person and the connection between the musculoskeletal system and disease and symptoms. (Ask. com)

Paralysis – loss of muscle function for one or more muscles. (Wikipedia)

Patent Medicine – a marketing technique, used in the United States for compounds promoted and sold as medical cures, which claimed the medicine had been "patented." In early England, medicines were given a "patent" of "Royal Favor." Often used to describe a Quack or cure-all medication.

Piles – also known as hemorrhoids, vascular structure in the anal canal that becomes inflamed. (Wikipedia)

Rheumatism – medical problems in the joints and connective tissue. A sub classification of arthritis. (Wikipedia)

Russian Steam – a steam bath often with mineral water. (Wikipedia)

Sanitarium – an older word for health resort, which provided fresh air, mineral waters, baths, and healthy food. In general, if spelled with "or" (Sanatorium), the facility most likely treated Tuberculosis. (*When There Were Poor Houses, Early Care in Rural New York, 1808–1950*)

Sciatica – A set of symptoms including pain that may be caused by general compression or irritation of one of five spinal nerve roots that give rise to each sciatic nerve. (Wikipedia)

Sitz Plunge – electro-thermal baths. (Wikipedia)

Sulphurous Springs (rotting egg smell) – a mineral spring in which the water contains sulphur or its compounds. (Oxford Dictionary)

Swedish Movement Cure – a series of systematic exercise therapeutically applied to the human body. (Wikipedia)

Torrent – a heavy uncontrolled outpouring. (Free Online Dictionary)

Turkish Bath – a type of steam bath with more water than steam. (Wikipedia)

Ulcerous Sores – a sore on the skin or mucous membranes. (Wikipedia)

Illustration and Photo Credits

Artists and Photographers
James Boles; Rachel Bridges; Danielle Herrmann;
Will Phillips; Melissa Royer.

Chapter 1
11: J. Boles, 2013. **15:** Orrin E. Dunlap Collection, Niagara
Falls Public Library, Local History Department, Niagara
Falls, New York. **17:** R. Bridges, 2013. **39:** R. Bridges, 2013.

Chapter 2
42: D. Herrmann, 2014. **47:** J. Boles, 2011. **55:** J. Boles,
2012.

Chapter 3
60: J. Boles, 2013. **70:** R. Bridges, 2013.

Chapter 4
87: R. Bridges, 2013. **95:** J. Boles, 2013. **101:** R. Bridges,
2014.

Chapter 5

108: M. Royer, 2012. **109:** M. Royer, 2012. **111:** M. Royer, 2012. **113:** J. Boles, 2013.

Chapter 6

120: R. Bridges, 2013. **122:** J. Boles, 2013.

Other photographs and images are from the archives of the Museum of disABILITY History in Buffalo, NY, and the files of James M Boles.

The Frontier House Timeline
1850–1959

Vedder House
Early 1850s: Built by the Vedder family
1854: Vedder House listed on a map of the town of Niagara
1855: Listed in a *Buffalo Daily Courier* newspaper ad

Globe Hotel
1857: Globe Hotel listed on a map of Niagara City
1860: Globe Hotel listed on a wall map of Niagara County

Frontier House
1875: Frontier House listed on a map of Suspension Bridge and in Beers' Atlas
1882: Listed in an advertisement for the *Complete Record of Niagara Falls and Vicinage*
1888: Listed in the *Suspension Bridge Directory* as a bath and specialty spring
1892: Listed again in *Niagara Falls and Vicinage* noting it's Sulphur Baths

Falls View Hotel

1902: Name was changed to Falls View Hotel with John L. Frank as proprietor

Frontier Hotel*

1908: Frontier Hotel listed on a map of Niagara Falls, Suspension Bridge

1909: John Pierce Langs listed as owner

*In a 1915 *Niagara Gazette* article, it refers to the Frontier House as the Frontier Hotel where John Scarupa was accused of running a disorderly house

Camel Hotel

1930: John Scarupa changed the name to Camel Hotel; it was listed as a dining and dancing hotel in the *Buffalo Express* paper

1953–1957: Dr. Richard Sherwood said that the structure will be remodeled to accommodate up-to-date business offices

1959: *Niagara Falls Gazette* reported some of the land still owned by the Langs' (John Pierce Lang being a descendant of a prominent physician of the village) would be taken over for construction of the Niagara parkway by the NY State Power Authority

Monteagle House/Hotel Timeline
2661 Lewiston Road/North Main Street Niagara Falls, New York

1848: Rocks taken from Niagara Gorge for erection of Monteagle Hotel

1855: Building completed (began 1848), built by the Niagara Suspension Bridge House Co.

1856 (January): International Railroad Bridge/Monteagle Festival

1856 (November): Opened for business under management of Charles B. Stuart

1857–1860: Mr. (Colonel) R. D. Cook "is having a large portion of the business"

1859: Sulphur Springs water introduced, bath houses erected in rear of hotel

1860: Messrs. Berry and Freeman (from Schenectady) took possession May 7th

1861–1868: Owned by Oscar DeCamp, managed by John Durnin

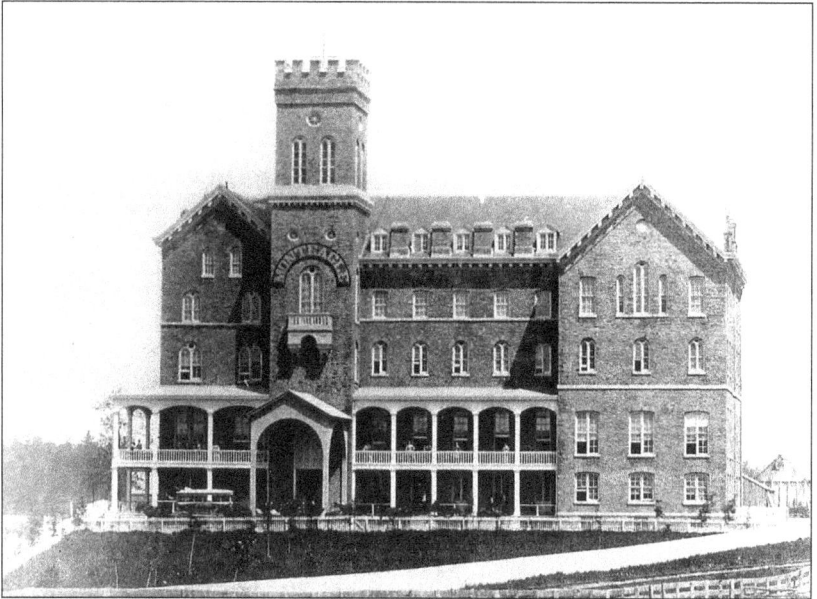

1865: Gas tank built (to supply north end of Niagara City/Falls Bellevue and Monteagle)

1868–1871: George and William P. Munro operate

1871–1873: David H. Tomlinson, Manager

1872: Listed for sale

1872–1874 and 1876-1877: J. Felix Nassoiy becomes owner

1874: Public auction, hotel and contents: May 20

1874: Tomlinson estate bought under foreclosure for $18,000 (November)

1875: Alexander & Terrill operate

1876 (April 6th): Foreclosure

1879: Alexian Brothers (Rev. Father Ignatius Sager) purchased for aged clergyman home

1881 (June): Auction sale

1882: Krapp, Kieffer and Smith, proprietors

1884 (July): Monteagle Hotel and Sanitarium by Dr. William R. Crumb

1885: John B. Manning's Mineral Springs Hotel

1886: Whirlpool Rapids Park opened on grounds, featuring C. D. Graham, rapids barrel runner

1887: Dr. Bell and Dr. Thompson, Niagara Springs Sanatorium

1888 (September): Willis & Burt Van Horn purchased from John B. Manning. Converted to cold storage house by Van Horn/Frank W. Stanley.

1889: VanHorns/Frank W. Stanley

1889: Suspension Bridge Cold Storage Warehouse (H. P. Stanley & Co.)

1906: Burt Van Horn takes over, upgrades cold storage

1922-1936: Cataract Ice Company (J. T. and W. H. Williamson)

1936: Slated to be razed

1937 (January): Burned by fire visible twenty miles distant

The Cataract House Timeline
1814–1945
(destroyed in a fire)

The Cataract House Hotel (aka River Parlors and Ballroom)

1814: Cataract House established

1855: Listed in a *Buffalo Daily Courier* newspaper ad

1868–1869: Alex Rivington Harris spoke about the hotel and it's strong-current baths

1871: Cataract House baths mentioned in an article in *Macmillan's Magazine*

1874: Cataract House baths listed for $.25 per ticket in the *Niagara Falls Gazette*

1877: Cataract House baths listed as the "admiration" of all those who enjoy them in *The Niagara Falls Gazette*

1882: Cataract House on a map by H. Wellge del. Beck & Pauli

1883: *The Niagara Falls Gazette* has an article about the Cataract House baths

1884: Cataract House listed in *Eighty-Eight Days in America* as having current baths

1945: Cataract House Destroyed by a fire

Tugby's, International Hotel, River Hotel, The Goat Island Hotel, The River Parlor Bath House, Behr Hotel

1857: An article states that Tugby's was turned into the International Hotel after the upper stories were finished off

1859: River Hotel is listed in a *Daily Gazette* article as being above the Cataract House

1860: A Niagara Falls business directory lists the River Hotel and Cataract House as *two separate* entities

1866: A Niagara County City Directory lists the Cataract House (Owned by Jerauld) and River hotel (Owned by Behr) as *two separate* entities

1885: When the River Hotel property was catalogued for purposes of the Niagara Reservation Commission in 1885, it was listed as "The Cataract Hotel Property, known as the River Parlors and Ball-Room-Sold."[6]

1927: An article in 1927, references the River Hotel as *its own entity*. This was referenced as a place where quiet and current baths were obtainable

1952: An article in 1952 references the Behr's River Hotel as an extension of the Cataract House. It boasts about the current baths that it offered patrons

Index

Books in the Vanishing Past Series:

When There Were Poorhouses: Early Care in Rural New York 1808 – 1950
by James M. Boles

No Harm was Done- Alternative Medicine in Lockport, New York
by James M. Boles

The Gold Cure Institutes of Niagara Falls, New York 1890s
by James M. Boles, EdD

Cures and Care in Niagara County, New York 1830-1950's

Stories from the Springs, The Niagara Frontier
by James M. Boles

No Harm Was Done-Alternative Medicine in Niagara Falls, New York
by James M. Boles